Urology

Editor

TODD J. DORAN

PHYSICIAN ASSISTANT CLINICS

www.physicianassistant.theclinics.com

Consulting Editor
JAMES A. VAN RHEE

January 2018 • Volume 3 • Number 1

ELSEVIER

1600 John F. Kennedy Boulevard • Suite 1800 • Philadelphia, Pennsylvania, 19103-2899

http://www.theclinics.com

PHYSICIAN ASSISTANT CLINICS Volume 3, Number 1
January 2018 ISSN 2405-7991, ISBN-13: 978-0-323-56649-0

Editor: Jessica McCool
Developmental Editor: Casey Potter

Physician Assistant Clinics (ISSN: 2405–7991) is published quarterly by Elsevier Inc., 360 Park Avenue South, New York, NY 10010-1710. Months of issue are January, April, July, and October. Periodicals postage paid at New York, NY and additional mailing offices. Subscription prices are $150.00 per year (US individuals), $205.00 (US institutions), $100.00 (US students), $150.00 (Canadian individuals), $257.00 (Canadian institutions), $100.00 (Canadian students), $150.00 (international individuals), $257.00 (international institutions), and $100.00 (international students). Foreign air speed delivery is included in all *Clinics* subscription prices. All prices are subject to change without notice. POSTMASTER: Send address changes to *Physician Assistant Clinics*, Elsevier Periodicals Customer Service, 11830 Westline Industrial Drive, St. Louis, MO 63146. Customer Service Health Sciences Division, Subscription Customer Service, 3251 Riverport Lane, Maryland Heights, MO 63043. **Customer Service: 1-800-654-2452 (U.S. and Canada); 314-447-8871 (outside U.S. and Canada). Fax: 314-447-8029. E-mail: journalscustomerservice-usa@elsevier.com (for print support); journalsonlinesupport-usa@elsevier.com (for online support).**

Reprints. For copies of 100 or more, of articles in this publication, please contact the Commercial Reprints Department, Elsevier Inc., 360 Park Avenue South, New York, NY 10010-1710. Tel. 212-633-3874; Fax: 212-633-3820; E-mail: reprints@elsevier.com.

Physician Assistant Clinics is covered in *MEDLINE/PubMed (Index Medicus)* and *EMBASE/Excerpta Medica, Current Contents/Clinical Medicine,* and *ISI/BIOMED. Physician Assistant Clinics* is indexed in ESCI.

PROGRAM OBJECTIVE
The goal of the *Physician Assistant Clinics* is to keep practicing physician assistants up to date with current clinical practice by providing timely articles reviewing the state of the art in patient care.

TARGET AUDIENCE
Physician Assistants and other healthcare professionals.

LEARNING OBJECTIVES
Upon completion of this activity, participants will be able to:
1. Review the management of various forms of urinary incontinence.
2. Discuss the management of common urinary concerns such as frequent UTI and kidney stones.
3. Recognize symptoms of male urinary issues such as lower urinary tract symptoms and erectile dysfunction.

ACCREDITATION
The Elsevier Office of Continuing Medical Education (EOCME) is accredited by the Accreditation Council for Continuing Medical Education (ACCME) to provide continuing medical education for physicians.

The EOCME designates this enduring material for a maximum of 15 *AMA PRA Category 1 Credit*(s)™. Physicians should claim only the credit commensurate with the extent of their participation in the activity.

All other health care professionals requesting continuing education credit for this enduring material will be issued a certificate of participation.

DISCLOSURE OF CONFLICTS OF INTEREST
The EOCME assesses conflict of interest with its instructors, faculty, planners, and other individuals who are in a position to control the content of CME activities. All relevant conflicts of interest that are identified are thoroughly vetted by EOCME for fair balance, scientific objectivity, and patient care recommendations. EOCME is committed to providing its learners with CME activities that promote improvements or quality in healthcare and not a specific proprietary business or a commercial interest.

The planning committee, staff, authors and editors listed below have identified no financial relationships or relationships to products or devices they or their spouse/life partner have with commercial interest related to the content of this CME activity:
Megan Rasmussen Bollner, MPAS, PA-C; Joseph Daniel; Todd J. Doran, EdD, PA-C, DFAAPA; Patrick Dougherty, MPAS, PA-C; Anjali Fortna; Brad Hornberger, MPAS, PA-C; Zain Z. Hyder, BS; Casey Jackson; Ryan Lewis, PA-C; Mark C. Lindgren, MD; Leah Logan; Jessica McCool; Kenneth A. Mitchell, MPAS, PA-C; Abby Moeller, PA-C; Jessica Nelson, MPAS, PA-C; Sanjay G. Patel, MD; Priyanka Tilak, PhD; Heidi Camus Turpen, MS, RD, MPAS, PA-C; James A. Van Rhee, MS, PA-C; Gwendolyn Brooke Zilinskas, MMS, PA-C.

The planning committee, staff, authors and editors listed below have identified financial relationships or relationships to products or devices they or their spouse/life partner have with commercial interest related to the content of this CME activity:
Michael Cookson, MD, MMHC is a consultant/advisor for Astellas Pharma US, Inc; Myovant Sciences; TesoRx Pharma, LLC; MDxHealth; Janssen Global Services, LLC; and Pacific Edge.

UNAPPROVED/OFF-LABEL USE DISCLOSURE
The EOCME requires CME faculty to disclose to the participants:
1. When products or procedures being discussed are off-label, unlabelled, experimental, and/or investigational (not US Food and Drug Administration [FDA] approved); and
2. Any limitations on the information presented, such as data that are preliminary or that represent ongoing research, interim analyses, and/or unsupported opinions. Faculty may discuss information about pharmaceutical agents that is outside of FDA-approved labelling. This information is intended solely for CME and is not intended to promote off-label use of these medications. If you have any questions, contact the medical affairs department of the manufacturer for the most recent prescribing information.

TO ENROLL
The CME program is available to all *Physician Assistant Clinics* subscribers at no additional fee. To subscribe to the *Physician Assistant Clinics*, call customer service at 1-800-654-2452 or sign up online at www.physicianassistant.theclinics.com.

METHOD OF PARTICIPATION

In order to claim credit, participants must complete the following:

1. Complete enrolment as indicated above.
2. Read the activity.
3. Complete the CME Test and Evaluation. Participants must achieve a score of 70% on the test. All CME Tests and Evaluations must be completed online.

CME INQUIRIES/SPECIAL NEEDS

For all CME inquiries or special needs, please contact elsevierCME@elsevier.com.

Contributors

CONSULTING EDITOR

JAMES A. VAN RHEE, MS, PA-C
Associate Professor, Program Director, Yale School of Medicine, Yale Physician Assistant Online Program, New Haven, Connecticut

EDITOR

TODD J. DORAN, EdD, PA-C, DFAAPA
Associate Professor, Division Chief, Program Director, Physician Associate Program, Department of Family and Preventive Medicine, The University of Oklahoma Health Sciences Center, College of Medicine, Oklahoma City, Oklahoma

AUTHORS

MEGAN RASMUSSEN BOLLNER, MPAS, PA-C
Department of Urology, The University of Texas Southwestern Medical Center, Dallas, Texas

MICHAEL COOKSON, MD, MMHC
Department of Urology, Stephenson Cancer Center, The University of Oklahoma Health Sciences Center, Oklahoma City, Oklahoma

TODD J. DORAN, EdD, PA-C, DFAAPA
Associate Professor, Division Chief, Program Director, Physician Associate Program, Department of Family and Preventive Medicine, The University of Oklahoma Health Sciences Center, College of Medicine, Oklahoma City, Oklahoma

PATRICK DOUGHERTY, MPAS, PA-C
Physician Assistant, Department of Urology, The University of Texas Southwestern Medical Center, Dallas, Texas

BRAD HORNBERGER, MPAS, PA-C
Faculty Associate, Department of Urology, The University of Texas Southwestern Medical Center, Dallas, Texas

ZAIN Z. HYDER, BS
The University of Oklahoma College of Medicine, Oklahoma City, Oklahoma

RYAN LEWIS, PA-C
Advanced Urology Associates, Joliet, Illinois

MARK C. LINDGREN, MD
Assistant Clinical Professor, Department of Urology, The University of Oklahoma, Oklahoma City, Oklahoma

KENNETH A. MITCHELL, MPAS, PA-C
Program Director, Meharry Medical College Physician Assistant Sciences Program,
Meharry Medical College, Nashville, Tennessee

ABBY MOELLER, PA-C
Department of Urology, Stephenson Cancer Center, The University of Oklahoma Health
Sciences Center, Oklahoma City, Oklahoma

JESSICA NELSON, MPAS, PA-C
Physician Assistant, Department of Urology, The University of Texas Southwestern
Medical Center, Dallas, Texas

SANJAY G. PATEL, MD
Assistant Professor, Department of Urology, Stephenson Cancer Center, The University
of Oklahoma Health Sciences Center, Oklahoma City, Oklahoma

PRIYANKA TILAK, PhD
Oncology Research Coordinator, Department of Urology, Stephenson Cancer Center,
The University of Oklahoma Health Sciences Center, Oklahoma City, Oklahoma

HEIDI CAMUS TURPEN, MS, RD, MPAS, PA-C
Physician Assistant, Urology Department, The University of Texas Southwestern Medical
Center, Dallas, Texas

GWENDOLYN BROOKE ZILINSKAS, MMS, PA-C
The University of Texas Southwestern Medical Center, Dallas, Texas

Contents

 Video content accompanies this article at http://www.
physicianassistant.theclinics.com.

Prostate cancer is the most common nonskin cancer in men in the United
States. Prostate-specific antigen (PSA) testing is the most common
method to stratify a man's risk of having prostate cancer. However, there
are well-established controversies and limitations to PSA testing. This
article addresses the risks and benefits of PSA screening. In addition, it
summarizes additional strategies to better determine a man's risk of having prostate cancer and the current guidelines from the American Urologic
Association and the National Comprehensive Cancer Network on PSA
testing.

Metastatic castrate-resistant prostate cancer (CRPC) is a disease state
characterized by a testosterone level of less than 50 ng/dL, with 2 consecutive increases in prostate-specific antigen (PSA) with a PSA level of
2 ng/dL or more. There have been several advances in the management
of CRPC. These therapies include immune therapy such as sipuleucel-T,
hormone therapies such as abiraterone acetate/prednisone or enzalutamide, radiation therapy such as radium-223, and chemotherapy such as
docetaxel and cabazitaxel. In addition to therapies directed toward treatment of prostate cancer, adjuvant therapies aimed at optimizing bone
health and quality of life in patients are also available.

Hematuria is defined as the presence of an abnormal quantity of red blood
cells in the urine and is categorized as microscopic or gross. Evaluation for
hematuria requires distinguishing glomerular (intrinsic renal disease
requiring nephrology evaluation) from nonglomerular (urinary tract disease
requiring urologic evaluation). The clinician must consider risk factors for
urinary tract malignancy and other mimics of hematuria to properly identify
the patient who needs further evaluation. Once confirmed, referral to a
urologist for evaluation with cross-sectional imaging, cystoscopy, and

possible urine cytology is required for timely diagnosis and treatment to prevent patient morbidity and mortality.

Overall prevalence of kidney stones is increasing as more stones are found incidentally on computed tomography and risk factors for stone disease (eg, obesity and type 2 diabetes mellitus) become more prevalent. Etiology of nephrolithiasis varies with stone type and depends on genetic, dietary, medication, lifestyle, and metabolic factors. Diagnostic evaluation of stone formers includes thorough history and physical, imaging, blood work, urinalysis, 24-hour urine collection, and analysis of stone fragments when possible. Medical management of stone disease includes increased hydration and dietary changes and/or pharmacologic therapy corresponding to an individual patient's metabolic derangements. Surgical treatment options for stone disease include shock wave lithotripsy, ureteroscopy, and percutaneous nephrolithotomy.

Urinary tract infections (UTIs) are among the most common bacterial infections, thus encountered by primary providers quite frequently. UTIs are classified as uncomplicated and complicated, which affects the duration of antibiotic treatment. Antibiotic stewardship is of the utmost important in treating infections to prevent development of bacterial resistance. Nonantibiotic treatment options in patients with UTIs should be considered. Asymptomatic bacteriuria should not be treated in nonpregnant individuals.

Urinary incontinence is a significant problem in health care today with a prevalence of up to 60% of women. It is also often underdiagnosed. However, by understanding the types of urinary incontinence (stress incontinence, urgency incontinence, mixed incontinence, overflow incontinence, and others) and the ways to take a focused history and perform an adequate physical examination, these patients can be diagnosed and treated with an array of medical and surgical therapies. These treatment options include oral medications for urgency urinary incontinence, nerve stimulation or Botulinum toxin for refractory patients or those who do not tolerate medication, and procedure-based therapies for stress incontinence. These procedures include pelvic floor physical therapy, urethral bulking, and sling procedures.

Physician assistants are vital in diagnosing and treating adult male patients with lower urinary tract symptoms. The evaluation and initiation of medical treatment often takes place in the primary care setting and medications titrated to the highest dosing or add-on therapy initiated. Patients refractory to medical treatment; who desire surgical opinion; and with probable urethral stricture disease, urinary retention, and abnormalities in the initial evaluation should be referred for urologic consultation. This article discusses the necessary history, physical examination, laboratory evaluation, limited special testing, initiation of medical treatment and appropriate follow-up, and when to obtain specialty consultation.

Neurogenic bladder (NGB) is a term used to describe lower urinary tract symptoms as a consequence of neurologic disease. The long-term effects of NGB can result in both lower and upper tract dysfunction and long-term renal damage. Discussed in this article are several diseases that contribute to neurologic voiding dysfunction. Also addressed are treatment and goals for patient management.

Erectile dysfunction (ED), although recognized as a pathologic condition for thousands of years, was not clearly defined until 1992, thus overcoming one of many barriers to treatment. ED is defined as the inability to achieve or maintain erection of sufficient rigidity and duration to permit satisfactory sexual performance. Causes of ED are psychogenic, vasculogenic, neurogenic, endocrinologic, cavernosal smooth muscle dysfunction, iatrogenic, pharmacologic, or combination of these. Diagnosis and evaluation of ED can be as simple as a questionnaire or involve complex testing and imaging. Treatment of ED follows a stepwise progression from noninvasive strategies to surgical placement of penile prostheses.

Physician assistants (PAs) commonly diagnose and treat men with hypogonadism in a urology practice. Challenges with the increasing prevalence of hypogonadism mandates that PAs have a clear understanding of the evaluation, treatment, and management. The lack of consensus among published guidelines adds to the challenge of conducting an appropriate evaluation. PAs must be familiar with the current guidelines for the treatment of hypogonadism. Careful consideration of the comorbidities is paramount for effective treatment and management of these patients. PAs must be familiar with the controversy surrounding initiating testosterone replacement therapy in hypogonadal men diagnosed with prostate cancer.

A male factor contribution to infertility is common. Ten percent to 15% of all couples attempting to conceive are infertile and half of these infertile couples have a male factor contribution. The proper initial workup for male factor infertility requires a thorough medical history, including medication use, and a complete physical examination, including genitalia, serum laboratory testing, and at least 2 complete semen analyses. Exogenous testosterone usage is a common modern cause or contributor to male infertility and can have a lasting impact on a man's fertility potential.

PHYSICIAN ASSISTANT CLINICS

THE CLINICS ARE AVAILABLE ONLINE!
Access your subscription at:
www.theclinics.com

Foreword

Recertification—Really?

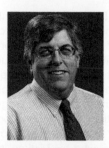

James A. Van Rhee, MS, PA-C
Consulting Editor

In the last issue, I discussed how *Physician Assistant Clinics* could be used to prepare for the PANCE and PANRE. That triggered a call from a colleague to discuss the need for recertification.

Should physician assistants (PA) have to recertify? If so, how often? I think everyone agrees we should have an initial certifying exam. But what about recertification exams? There are definitely two sides to this. On the one hand, no one likes to take time out of their busy practice to study for a general exam. Many PAs feel they are knowledgeable in their area of practice, provide excellent care, and patients are happy; so why take an exam? The PA practicing in a specialty area has to wonder why they take a generalist exam to continue to practice in their specialty area. What about all the discussion: does recertifying improve patient care and outcomes?

We should recertify, but we should have options. As advocates for life-long learning, it is one of the profession's professional competencies. We need to show we are engaged in learning and willing to be evaluated on it, not because it improves patient care (jury is out on that), but because it's the right thing for us as life-long learners. But provide options. Everyone should retest with the generalist exam six years after graduating. We should all be aware of how to treat and manage diabetes and hypertension, for example. After this second generalist exam, now the options open up. What to recertify by exam? The generalist exam should be available online, both to take home and at a testing center. Want to take a specialty exam, in place of the generalist exam, to show you have added knowledge? Sure. It too should be available online, both to take home and at a testing center. Now the twist; if we are really interested in life-long learning, then the exam has to provide us with feedback. We need explanations and references so we can update our knowledge. The exam must be up-to-date and test practical, everyday knowledge. If we are really doing the CME and reading (like *Physician Assistant Clinics*), as we say we are, a test like this should be straightforward and enhance our knowledge. The exam should not be punitive. If you fail after

Physician Assist Clin 3 (2018) xiii–xiv
https://doi.org/10.1016/j.cpha.2017.10.002
2405-7991/18/© 2017 Published by Elsevier Inc.

two attempts, other options should be available for you to maintain your certification while you review material and get ready for retesting.

Let's not remove recertification by examination to maintain certification just because other professions don't or just because it's hard. Let's do it because it's right for us as health care providers to let others and ourselves know we are life-long learners and that we want to assess this life-long learning.

In this issue, we are focusing on urology. Guest editor Todd Doran has put together an excellent issue covering a wide variety of topics. Doran himself provides an excellent review on lower urinary tract symptoms, and with Tilak and others, a discussion of the evaluation and workup of hematuria. Turpen provides us with the latest in frequent urinary tract infections. We have a couple of articles on prostate cancer. Lewis provides a review of prostate cancer screening, and Moeller reviews metastatic castrate-resistant prostate cancer. A variety of male disorders are discussed. Lindgren reviews male infertility; Dougherty discusses erectile dysfunction, and Mitchell looks at hypogonadism. Hornberger and Rasmussen Bollner cover kidney stones, a topic near and dear to my heart. Female urinary incontinence is reviewed by Zilinkas, and Nelson provides a discussion of neurogenic bladder and its management.

I hope you enjoy the ninth issue of *Physician Assistant Clinics*. Our next issue will provide you with a review of the latest in otolaryngology.

James A. Van Rhee, MS, PA-C
Yale School of Medicine
Yale Physician Assistant Online Program
100 Church Street South, Suite A230
New Haven, CT 06519, USA

E-mail address:
james.vanrhee@yale.edu

Website:
http://www.paonline.yale.edu

Preface
Plumbing Department on Aisle 2

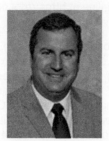

Todd J. Doran, EdD, PA-C, DFAAPA
Editor

 Video content accompanies this article at http://www.physicianassistant.
theclinics.com.

Most of us fear the prospect of tackling electrical or plumbing problems in our home, and my experience is we feel the same way when dealing with urologic or neurologic problems in the office (Video 1). Plumbing (urologic) and electrical (neurologic) problems are usually unrelated in your home, but oftentimes they are related in a patient, and assessing the septic (colorectal) system is clinically pertinent. The purpose of this journal special issue is to lessen the fear of the primary care Physician Assistant (PA) to tackle routine urologic problems that most commonly can be managed medically. For the specialist, it is a welcome event to see a referred patient who has been adequately evaluated and appropriate medications tried at sufficient doses and duration to assess for a response. The purpose of a urologic surgery consult is to determine if the patient needs an operation. It is impossible to do that efficiently if a patient hasn't failed medical management nor has been sufficiently evaluated.

I personally hand-picked each author and topic from the perspective of the types of urologic problems I've encountered in a tertiary academic health center over the past twenty years. The authors assembled have many years of urologic specialty experience at tertiary referral centers, and they in turn work with seasoned fellowship-trained urologists. Their perspective and advice are grounded in evidence-based practice and clinical guidelines established by scientific evidence and key opinion. The reader will improve their ability to manage the most common adult conditions referred to urologic surgery: male infertility, prostate cancer screening, advanced prostate cancer, hematuria, kidney stones, frequent urinary tract infections, female urinary incontinence, male lower urinary tract symptoms, erectile dysfunction, hypogonadism, and neurogenic bladder. It is impossible to cover them all, but this is a good primer.

I want to thank all of the contributors for their efforts in sharing their expertise on paper in a way to lessen the anxiety of the primary care PA being able to tackle the

Physician Assist Clin 3 (2018) xv–xvi
https://doi.org/10.1016/j.cpha.2017.10.001
2405-7991/18/© 2017 Elsevier Inc. All rights reserved.

problems presented here. Thank you for hanging out with us on aisle 2, and we hope you learned at least three new things to take back with you into practice.

SUPPLEMENTARY DATA

Supplementary data related to this article can be found online at https://doi.org/10.1016/j.cpha.2017.10.001.

Todd J. Doran, EdD, PA-C, DFAAPA
Physician Associate Program
Department of Family and Preventive Medicine
College of Medicine
The University of Oklahoma Health Sciences Center
940 Stanton L. Young Boulevard, Suite 357
Oklahoma City, OK 73104, USA

E-mail address:
doranohana@gmail.com

Prostate Cancer Screening

Ryan Lewis, PA-C

KEYWORDS

- Prostate-specific antigen testing • PSA screening • Shared decision-making
- Elevated PSA

KEY POINTS

- A clinician and patient should engage in shared decision-making before engaging in prostate-specific antigen (PSA) testing.
- The PSA test is the most common method to determine a man's risk of having prostate cancer, but it is not cancer specific.
- There are additional tests beyond the PSA test to stratify a man's risk of having prostate cancer.

OVERVIEW

Prostate cancer is the most common nonskin cancer in men in the United States with approximately 1 in 7 men developing prostate cancer, and it is the third leading cause of cancer death in men.[1] In 1994, the US Food and Drug Administration (FDA) approved the use of prostate-specific antigen (PSA) screening to test asymptomatic men for prostate cancer and, since implementation, the incidence of metastasis and mortality from prostate cancer have significantly decreased.[2,3] However, the use of PSA screening for prostate cancer has its limitations. Although it is very prostate-specific it is not cancer-specific. Other factors besides prostate cancer, such as an enlarged prostate or prostatitis, can cause an elevated PSA. In addition, PSA levels serve as a continuum in which the risk of prostate cancer increases with increasing PSA, but there is no level of PSA below which the risk of prostate cancer can be eliminated. Even though prostate cancer is very common, a man only has a 2.6% risk of dying from it because most cases of prostate cancer are slow growing and may never cause morbidity or mortality.[4]

CONTROVERSIES OF PROSTATE-SPECIFIC ANTIGEN TESTING

There is criticism that prostate cancer is overdiagnosed and overtreated in the United States. Numerous studies have been conducted to try to quantify the mortality benefits of PSA screening. Although it is known that PSA testing leads to a higher incidence

Disclosure Statement: The author has no disclosures with any commercial or financial conflicts of interests, and the author has no funding sources.
Advanced Urology Associates, 1541 Riverboat Center Drive, Joliet, IL 60431, USA
E-mail address: rglewis23@gmail.com

of cancer detection, it is unknown whether the increased detection is accompanied by a significant reduction in mortality that also outweighs the harms of overdetection and overtreatment. The Prostate, Lung, Colorectal, and Ovarian (PLCO) Cancer Screening Trial and the European Randomized Study of Screening for Prostate Cancer (ERSPC) are the most commonly referenced studies in the literature regarding this issue. Although the PLCO trial demonstrated no benefit from PSA screening, the trial had flaws, such as a high contamination rate, and a reanalysis published in the *New England Journal of Medicine* in 2016 confirmed that.[5] The ERSPC trial demonstrated a significant prostate cancer mortality benefit with PSA screening, but it is unknown whether the benefit outweighed the harms of screening that can lead to the overdiagnosis and overtreatment of prostate cancer. These were the 2 main studies the US Preventive Services Task Force (USPSTF) used when they gave a grade D recommendation against screening for prostate cancer in May 2012, which caused a great deal of controversy.[6] However, the USPSTF revised their recommendation in 2017 giving PSA screening a grade C for men ages 55 to 69 years and maintained their grade D recommendation for men ages 70 years and older.[7]

GUIDELINES

Two organizations, the American Urological Association (AUA) and the National Comprehensive Cancer Network (NCCN), have guidelines to help clinicians use PSA testing (**Table 1**). Shared decision-making with the patient is a concept that holds true throughout all prostate cancer detection guidelines. A patient must know the risks, benefits, and alternatives of prostate cancer screening before making an informed decision. Even though the AUA and NCCN have put forth guidelines for clinicians it must be remembered that guidelines are no substitute for clinical judgment or experience. With all the confusion surrounding PSA testing, it can be difficult to determine the best course of action for a patient. However, an excellent place to start is to recognize the inherent strengths and weaknesses of the USPSTF recommendations. Second, it is important to engage in shared decision-making with the patient. Third, identify the patients who will likely benefit the most from screening based on risk factors, such as age 55 to 69 years, African American race, and family history of prostate cancer. Fourth, consider a baseline PSA test between the ages of 45 to 54 years. A higher PSA in midlife is associated with a higher risk of future prostate cancer and this baseline value can help stratify a patient's risk to better determine frequency of testing.[8,9] Finally, refer to a health care provider who specializes in urology when faced with a confirmed elevated PSA, an abnormally rising PSA, an abnormal digital rectal examination (DRE), or a patient with significant risk factors. There are new and emerging tests available to better stratify a patient's risk of having or dying from prostate cancer, such as biomarkers, genomic testing, and multiparametric MRI. Collaboration between the patient, clinicians in primary care, and urology is paramount to optimize patient outcomes.

MANAGING AN ELEVATED PROSTATE-SPECIFIC ANTIGEN

The half-life of PSA is approximately 3 days, so when encountering an abnormal PSA test it is prudent to repeat the test 1 month later for confirmation.[10,11] One study demonstrated that approximately 25% of men with an initial PSA between 4 and 10 ng/mL had normal PSA levels on repeat testing.[12] Also, when facing an elevated PSA in an asymptomatic man, the AUA, as part of the Choosing Wisely campaign, recommends against prescribing a course of antibiotics before rechecking a PSA value because there is a lack of clinical studies to show that antibiotics actually decrease PSA levels in

Table 1
Guidelines for PSA testing from the American Urologic Association and the National Comprehensive Cancer Network

Recommendations	AUA[a]	NCCN[b]
Shared decision-making	Yes	Yes
Age to offer screening in average-risk patient	55	45
Age to offer screening in high-risk patient	<55	45
Interval of screening	2 y but should be individualized based on risk factors and PSA value	Individualized If PSA <1 every 2–4 y If PSA 1–3 every 1–2 y If PSA confirmed >3 consider repeating in 6–12 mo, biomarkers, or biopsy
Age to stop screening	70 or <10–15 y life expectancy Some men >70 in excellent health may benefit from screening	75 or <10 y life expectancy A very select group >75 in excellent health may benefit from screening
Digital rectal examination	Lack of evidence as primary screening tool May be useful in men with an elevated PSA	May be performed in asymptomatic men along with a PSA after shared decision-making Perform in all men with an abnormal PSA

[a] Detection of Prostate Cancer: American Urological Association. Auanetorg. 2013. Available at: https://www.auanet.org/education/guidelines/prostate-cancer-detection.cfm. Accessed May 22, 2016.
[b] Prostate Cancer Early Detection. NCCN Clinical Practice Guidelines in Oncology. 2016. Available at: https://www.nccn.org/professionals/physician_gls/pdf/prostate_detection.pdf. Accessed May 22, 2016.

asymptomatic men and that a decrease in PSA does not indicate the absence of prostate cancer.[13–15] Most men with an elevated PSA do not have prostate cancer. In fact, only about 25% of men with a PSA value between 4 and 10 ng/mL have a positive biopsy.[16] However, there is no level of PSA below which the risk of prostate cancer can be eliminated. One trial demonstrated that 15% of men with a PSA level below 4 ng/mL had prostate cancer.[17] This has led to further studies that have investigated lowering the PSA cutoff to avoid missing men with prostate cancer who have PSA values below 4 ng/mL.[18–20] However, although lowering the PSA cutoff would improve test sensitivity, a lower PSA cutoff would also reduce specificity leading to far more false-positive tests and unnecessary biopsies. Although the NCCN recommends a total PSA cutoff of 3 ng/mL, a cutoff of 4 ng/mL has been the accepted standard because it is thought to balance the tradeoff between detecting important cancers at a curable stage and avoiding the detection of clinically insignificant disease. Therefore, there is a need to be aware of additional methods and tests beyond the PSA to better stratify a man's risk of having prostate cancer because having a normal or abnormal PSA value does not necessarily mean a man can avoid a biopsy or immediately needs one.

BEYOND THE PROSTATE-SPECIFIC ANTIGEN TEST

The AUA acknowledges that the literature supporting the efficacy of tests other than the PSA test is limited. Although some data suggest use of these secondary screening tools may reduce unnecessary biopsies while still maintaining the ability to detect aggressive prostate cancer, more research is needed to confirm this.[21] The NCCN addresses these additional tests and methods individually and then makes a recommendation based on the evidence that is currently available.[22]

DIGITAL RECTAL EXAMINATION

The AUA and NCCN do not recommend the DRE as a stand-alone primary screening test. It may be considered in addition to PSA testing after a risk-benefit discussion is had to help determine the need for a prostate biopsy. Those with an abnormal DRE should be considered for a prostate biopsy even with a normal PSA because it may identify high-grade cancers in such situations. The NCCN believes that a DRE should be performed in all men with an abnormal PSA.

AGE-SPECIFIC REFERENCE RANGES

PSA levels increase with age, largely due to a higher prevalence of an enlarged prostate. Thus, rather than rely on a single reference range for men of all age groups, it may be more appropriate to have age-specific reference ranges to make the PSA test a more discriminating tumor marker to find more potentially curable cancers in younger men and to detect only clinically significant cancers in older men. Therefore, for better discriminating power, it has been proposed to adjust the cutoff range to 2.5 ng/mL in men aged 40 to 49 years, to 3.5 ng/mL in men 50 to 59 years, to 4.5 ng/mL in men aged 60 to 69 years, and to 6.5 ng/mL in men aged 70 to 79 years.[23] Age-specific cutoffs have been investigated with equivocal results; however, 2 of the largest such studies concluded that a PSA cutoff of 4 ng/mL across all age groups best preserves the balance between risks, benefits, sensitivity, and specificity.[24,25] The NCCN makes no recommendations regarding the routine use of this practice because the exact role of age-specific PSA cutoffs is still unclear.

PROSTATE-SPECIFIC ANTIGEN VELOCITY

The rate of change in PSA over time is termed PSA velocity (PSAV) and is determined by at least 3 separate PSA values calculated over at least an 18-month period. A PSAV of 0.35 ng/mL per year increase for PSA values less than 4 ng/mL and 0.75 ng/mL per year increase for PSA values greater than 4 ng/mL are typically the values referred to when discussing PSAV.[26] The use of PSAV has been extensively studied but with mixed results and inconsistencies regarding the exact cutoffs for PSAV.[27–29] However, a systematic review of the literature involving 87 articles up to 2007 found that PSAV adds little to the diagnostic accuracy provided by PSA alone.[30] In addition, a retrospective analysis of data from The Prostate Cancer Prevention Trial, a large prostate cancer screening trial, suggested that incorporating PSAV only led to a very small enhancement in the predictive accuracy of detecting prostate cancer.[31] Most panelists on the NCCN committee agree that a PSAV of greater than 0.35 ng/mL per year for men with low PSA values is only 1 criterion to consider when deciding whether to perform a biopsy. Panelists do not agree on the threshold of PSAV that should prompt consideration of biopsy, but PSAV may aid in the decision-making process. However, other factors, such as total PSA, age, race, family history, and comorbidities, should be considered first.

FREE PROSTATE-SPECIFIC ANTIGEN

Free PSA, expressed as a ratio of total PSA, has the potential to improve the detection of prostate cancer. The FDA has approved the use of free PSA for the early detection of prostate cancer in men with normal prostate examinations and PSA levels between 4 ng/mL and 10 ng/mL. Numerous studies have shown that the percentage of free PSA is significantly lower in men who have prostate cancer compared with men who do not.[16,32] In 1 study, 56% of men with a free PSA less than 10% had prostate cancer, whereas only 8% of men with a free PSA greater than 25% had prostate cancer. However, a large meta-analysis of the diagnostic performance of free PSA demonstrated that it is a useful adjunct to a total PSA value under certain conditions and it may assist clinical decision-making only when levels reach extreme values.[33] Although there is no agreement on the best threshold value for free PSA, values below 10% raise suspicion for prostate cancer and values above 25% can reliably predict the absence of clinically significant prostate cancer. The NCCN recommends clinicians to consider performing a free PSA in men with a PSA greater than 3 ng/mL who have not yet had a biopsy.

PROSTATE HEALTH INDEX

The prostate health index (PHI) is a blood test that is a combination of total PSA, free PSA, and proPSA (precursor to PSA). It is FDA-approved for use in men with PSA values between 4 and 10 ng/mL. In a large multicenter study it was found to have better sensitivity and specificity than total PSA and free PSA for cancer detection in men with PSA values between 2 and 10 ng/mL.[34] It has the potential to reduce negative biopsies by 36% with very few aggressive cancers missed when the PHI cutoff is 24.[35] The NCCN recommends considering the PHI in making biopsy decisions for men with PSA levels between 3 and 10 ng/mL.

4KSCORE

The 4Kscore is a blood test that incorporates total PSA, free PSA, intact PSA, and human kallikrein 2 (hK2). The test reports the percent likelihood from 1% to 95% of finding high-grade cancer (Gleason 7 or greater) on a prostate biopsy. A multicenter clinical utility study found a 65% reduction in prostate biopsies using the 4Kscore.[36] The NCCN recommends 4Kscore be considered in men with a PSA greater than 3 ng/mL to provide an estimate of the probability of high-grade prostate cancer on a biopsy; however, because no cutoff threshold has been established that should trigger a biopsy, the results of the test should be discussed with the patient about whether to proceed with a biopsy.

RISK CALCULATORS

Prostate cancer risk calculators have been developed to estimate a man's risk for prostate cancer using multiple factors, such as age, family history, race, DRE, PSA, and previous biopsy results. One of the most widely used calculators is the Prostate Cancer Prevention Trial Risk Calculator 2.0 and it is free to use online.[37] It has been externally validated and assists in determining the risk of low-grade versus high-grade disease on biopsy. However, no percentage of cutoff points to trigger a biopsy has been established and the NCCN does not recommend the use of risk calculators alone to determine whether a biopsy is indicated.

IMAGING TECHNIQUES

Imaging modalities, specifically multiparametric MRI, for selecting those who need a prostate biopsy or to allow for lesion-specific biopsies are becoming more widely used. However, the current data do not conclusively support its use for determining which men should undergo an initial prostate biopsy.[38–40] The NCCN recommends that an MRI alone not be used to decide whether to initially biopsy, and that a negative MRI is not an indication to forego a biopsy. However, the NCCN states an MRI or MRI-guided targeted biopsy should be considered in a repeat biopsy setting.

SUMMARY

It is important that a clinician and patient engage in shared decision-making before proceeding with PSA screening. In addition, one must understand that prostate cancer can be present when the PSA is below 4 and is still statistically more likely to be absent when the PSA is above 4. When encountering an elevated PSA, one should look for factors other than cancer that may have caused this elevated value, such as prostatitis, an enlarged prostate, or recent urethral instrumentation. In addition, it is important to know whether a patient is taking a 5-alpha reductase inhibitor (5-ARI) because this class of drugs lowers the PSA by approximately 50% after 6 months, yet has no effect on free PSA.[41,42] Also, if a patient is placed on a 5-ARI and the PSA does not decline by approximately 50% or it steadily rises, there should be suspicion for prostate cancer. Once secondary causes of an elevated PSA have been considered, the PSA should be repeated approximately 4 weeks later, preferably using the same laboratory. Antibiotics should not be prescribed in the interim unless a man has signs or symptoms of prostatitis. Once a PSA of 4 ng/mL or greater is confirmed, it is recommended to offer these men a prostate biopsy. If a clinician or patient would like more information on the risk of having prostate cancer before undergoing a biopsy, the evidence supports the use of obtaining a free PSA or the PHI to better determine a man's risk of having prostate cancer. The 4Kscore can also be used in men who have an elevated PSA to predict the likelihood of having low-grade or high-grade cancer on biopsy. PSAV and online risk calculators are strategies that may assist in clinical decision-making, but the evidence does not support their use alone in determining which men should undergo biopsy. Future improvement, research, and cost analysis is needed on the role of MRI to determine which men should undergo an initial biopsy; however, it has proven very useful in certain settings, such as a rising PSA with a previous negative biopsy and for men diagnosed with prostate cancer who are on active surveillance.[43]

REFERENCES

1. What are the key statistics about prostate cancer? American Cancer Society; 2016. Available at: http://www.cancer.org/cancer/prostatecancer/detailedguide/prostate-cancer-key-statistics. Accessed May 10, 2017.
2. Stanford JL, Stephenson RA, Coyle LM, et al. Prostate cancer trends 1973-1995, SEER program, National Cancer Institute. Bethesda (MD): NIH Pub; 1998.
3. Paquette E, Sun L, Paquette L, et al. Improved prostate cancer-specific survival and other disease parameters: impact of prostate-specific antigen testing. Urology 2002;60(5):756–9.
4. Lifetime risk of developing or dying from cancer. Cancerorg; 2016. Available at: http://www.cancer.org/cancer/cancerbasics/lifetime-probability-of-developing-or-dying-from-cancer. Accessed May 10, 2017.
5. Shoag J, Mittal S, Hu J. Reevaluating PSA testing rates in the PLCO trial. N Engl J Med 2016;374(18):1795–6.
6. Final Recommendation Statement: prostate cancer: screening. US Preventive Services Task Force; 2016. Available at: http://www.uspreventiveservicestaskforce.org/Page/Document/RecommendationStatementFinal/prostate-cancer-screening. Accessed May 25, 2017.

7. Prostate cancer screening draft recommendations. U.S. Preventive Services Task Force; 2017. Available at: https://screeningforprostatecancer.org/. Accessed May 25, 2017.

8. Ulmert D, Cronin A, Björk T, et al. Prostate-specific antigen at or before age 50 as a predictor of advanced prostate cancer diagnosed up to 25 years later: a case-control study. BMC Med 2008;6(1):6.

9. Kovac E, Carlsson S, Lilja H, et al. Baseline PSA before age 60 as a predictor of important prostate cancer diagnosis and prostate cancer-specific mortality in the intervention arm of the prostate, lung, colorectal and ovarian trial. J Urol 2016; 195(4):445–6.

10. Nixon RG, Wener MH, Smith KM, et al. Biological variation of prostate specific antigen levels in serum: an evaluation of day-to-day physiological fluctuations In a well-defined cohort of 24 patients. J Urol 1997;157:2183.

11. Eastham JA, Riedel E, Scardino PT, et al. Variation of serum prostate-specific antigen levels: an evaluation of year-to-year fluctuations. JAMA 2003;289:2695.

12. Lavallee LT, Binette A, Witiuk K, et al. Reducing the harm of prostate cancer screening: repeated prostate-specific antigen testing. Mayo Clin Proc 2016;91: 17–22.

13. Heldwein FL, Teloken PE, Hartmann AA, et al. Antibiotics and observation have a similar impact on asymptomatic patients with a raised PSA. BJU Int 2011;107(10): 1576–81.

14. Stopiglia RM, Ferreira U, Silva MM Jr, et al. Prostate specific antigen decrease and prostate cancer diagnosis: antibiotic versus placebo prospective randomized clinical trial. J Urol 2010;183(3):940–5.

15. "Don't treat an elevated PSA with antibiotics for patients not experiencing other symptoms." Choosing Wisely. American Urological Association; 2013. Available at: http://www.choosingwisely.org/clinician-lists/american-urological-association-treating-elevated-psa-with-antibiotics/. Accessed May 25, 2017.

16. Catalona WJ, Partin AW, Slawin KM, et al. Use of the percentage of free prostate-specific antigen to enhance differentiation of prostate cancer from benign prostatic disease: a prospective multicenter clinical trial. JAMA 1998;279:1542–7.

17. Thompson IM, Pauler DK, Goodman PJ, et al. Prevalence of prostate cancer among men with a prostate-specific antigen level < or =4.0 ng per milliliter. N Engl J Med 2004;350:2239–46.

18. Catalona WJ, Smith DS, Ornstein DK. Prostate cancer detection in men with serum PSA concentrations of 2.6 to 4.0 ng/mL and benign prostate examination. Enhancement of specificity with free PSA measurements. JAMA 1997; 277:1452.

19. Babaian RJ, Johnston DA, Naccarato W, et al. The incidence of prostate cancer in a screening population with a serum prostate specific antigen between 2.5 and 4.0 ng/ml: relation to biopsy strategy. J Urol 2001;165:757.

20. Gilbert SM, Cavallo CB, Kahane H, et al. Evidence suggesting PSA cutpoint of 2.5 ng/mL for prompting prostate biopsy: review of 36,316 biopsies. Urology 2005;65:549.

21. Carter HB, Albertsen PC, Barry MJ, et al. Early detection of prostate cancer: AUA Guideline. J Urol 2013;190:419–26.

22. National Comprehensive Cancer Network. Prostate Cancer Early Detection. Available at: https://www.nccn.org/professionals/physician_gls/pdf/prostate_detection.pdf. Accessed May 25, 2017.

23. Oesterling JE, Jacobsen SJ, Chute CG, et al. Serum prostate-specific antigen in a community-based population of healthy men. Establishment of age-specific reference ranges. JAMA 1993;270:860–4.

24. Catalona WJ, Hudson MA, Scardino PT, et al. Selection of optimal prostate specific antigen cutoffs for early detection of prostate cancer: receiver operating characteristic curves. J Urol 1994;152:2037.

25. Morgan TO, Jacobsen SJ, McCarthy WF, et al. Age-specific reference ranges for prostate-specific antigen in black men. N Engl J Med 1996;335:304–10.

26. Carter HB, Pearson JD, Metter EJ, et al. Longitudinal evaluation of prostate-specific antigen levels in men with and without prostate disease. JAMA 1992; 267:2215–20. Available at: http://www.ncbi.nlm.nih.gov/pubmed/1372942.

27. Carter HB, Ferrucci L, Kettermann A, et al. Detection of life-threatening prostate cancer with prostate-specific antigen velocity during a window of curability. J Natl Cancer Inst 2006;98:1521–7.

28. D'Amico AV, Chen MH, Roehl KA, et al. Preoperative PSA velocity and the risk of death from prostate cancer after radical prostatectomy. N Engl J Med 2004;351: 125–35.

29. D'Amico AV, Renshaw AA, Sussman B, et al. Pretreatment PSA velocity and risk of death from prostate cancer following external beam radiation therapy. JAMA 2005;294:440–7.

30. Vickers AJ, Savage C, O'Brien MF, et al. Systematic review of pretreatment prostate-specific antigen velocity and doubling time as predictors for prostate cancer. J Clin Oncol 2009;27:398.

31. Vickers AJ, Wolters T, Savage CJ, et al. Prostate-specific antigen velocity for early detection of prostate cancer: result from a large, representative, population-based cohort. Eur Urol 2009;56:753.

32. Partin AW, Brawer MK, Subong EN, et al. Prospective evaluation of percent free-PSA and complexed-PSA for early detection of prostate cancer. Prostate Cancer Prostatic Dis 1998;1:197–203.

33. Lee R, Localio AR, Armstrong K, et al. A meta-analysis of the performance characteristics of the free prostate-specific antigen test. Urology 2006;67:762.

34. Catalona WJ, Partin AW, Sanda MG, et al. A multicenter study of [-2]pro-prostate specific antigen combined with prostate specific antigen and free prostate specific antigen for prostate cancer detection in the 2.0 to 10.0 ng/ml prostate specific antigen range. J Urol 2011;185:1650–5.

35. de la Calle C, Patil D, Wei JT, et al. Multicenter evaluation of the Prostate Health Index to detect aggressive prostate cancer in biopsy naive men. J Urol 2015;194: 65–72.

36. Konety B, Zappala SM, Parekh DJ, et al. The 4Kscore(R) test reduces prostate biopsy rates in community and academic urology practices. Rev Urol 2015;17: 231–40.

37. Ankerst DP, Hoefler J, Bock S, et al. The Prostate Cancer Prevention Trial Risk Calculator 2.0 for the prediction of low- versus high-grade prostate cancer. Urology 2014;83(6):1362–7.

38. Kuru TH, Roethke MC, Seidenader J, et al. Critical evaluation of magnetic resonance imaging targeted, transrectal ultrasound guided transperineal fusion biopsy for detection of prostate cancer. J Urol 2013;190:1380–6.

39. Lamb BW, Tan WS, Rehman A, et al. Is prebiopsy MRI good enough to avoid prostate biopsy? A cohort study over a 1-year period. Clin Genitourin Cancer 2015;13:512–7.

40. Tonttila PP, Lantto J, Paakko E, et al. Prebiopsy multiparametric magnetic resonance imaging for prostate cancer diagnosis in biopsy-naive men with suspected prostate cancer based on elevated prostate-specific antigen values: results from a randomized prospective blinded controlled trial. Eur Urol 2015;69(3):419–25.
41. Roehrborn CG, Boyle P, Nickel JC, et al. Efficacy and safety of a dual inhibitor of 5-alpha-reductase types 1 and 2 (dutasteride) in men with benign prostatic hyperplasia. Urology 2002;60:434–41.
42. Pannek J, Marks LS, Pearson JD, et al. Influence of finasteride on free and total serum prostate specific antigen levels in men with benign prostatic hyperplasia. J Urol 1998;159:449–53.
43. Bjurlin MA, Mendhiratta N, Wysock JS, et al. Multiparametric MRI and targeted prostate biopsy: Improvements in cancer detection, localization, and risk assessment. Cent European J Urol 2016;69(1):9–18.

Metastatic Castrate-Resistant Prostate Cancer Practical Review

Abby Moeller, PA-C*, Michael Cookson, MD, MMHC,
Sanjay G. Patel, MD

KEYWORDS

- Castrate-resistant prostate cancer • CRPC • Androgen deprivation therapy • ADT
- LHRH • Immune therapy • Skeletal-related event (SRE)

KEY POINTS

- Androgen deprivation therapy, with goals of creating a castrate-level testosterone, is the primary baseline treatment of metastatic prostate cancer and should be continued indefinitely.
- There are many different therapies now available for men with metastatic castrate-resistant prostate cancer (CRPC). Optimal selection of each therapy depends on the patient's clinical assessment and performance status.
- In addition to treatment of metastatic disease, attention should also be directed toward therapies that optimize the patient's bone health and quality of life.

DEFINITIONS

Castrate: serum total testosterone level of less than 50 ng/dL.[1]

Castrate-resistant prostate cancer (CRPC): patient with prostate cancer that has an increasing PSA level or worsening radiographic changes in the face of a total testosterone level of less than 50 ng/dL.[2]

Hormone-sensitive prostate cancer: patient with prostate cancer and a detectable PSA level that is stable or decreasing despite androgen deprivation therapy (ADT).

Metastasis: visible signs of cancer on imaging, beyond the primary cancer.

Prostate-specific antigen (PSA): enzyme secreted from prostate epithelial cells.[3]

Funding: None.
Department of Urology, Stephenson Cancer Center, The University of Oklahoma Health Sciences Center, 800 North East 10th Street, Suite 4300, Oklahoma City, OK 73104, USA
* Corresponding author.
E-mail address: Abby-Moeller@ouhsc.edu

Physician Assist Clin 3 (2018) 11–21
http://dx.doi.org/10.1016/j.cpha.2017.08.003
2405-7991/18/© 2017 Elsevier Inc. All rights reserved.

INTRODUCTION

Prostate cancer remains the most commonly diagnosed malignancy in men and is diagnosed and monitored using serum PSA.[4] Patients with prostate cancer are broadly categorized as having localized or metastatic disease. Patients diagnosed with localized prostate cancer typically undergo primary treatment with cryotherapy, radiation therapy, or surgery and should have a persistently undetectable or stable low PSA, which indicates treatment success. It is recommended to follow the PSA for at least 20 years after primary therapy because increases in PSA indicate primary treatment failure and may necessitate further adjuvant therapies.[5] A small subset of patients who undergo primary treatment undergo disease progression and develop metastatic disease. Patients initially diagnosed with metastatic disease or who progress to metastatic disease after primary treatment have increasing and often markedly elevated levels of PSA.[6]

The mainstay treatment of patients with metastatic prostate cancer is lifelong ADT. ADT aims to lower the total testosterone (T) level to castrate levels, defined as less than 50 ng/dL. ADT can be accomplished through surgical castration (bilateral orchiectomy) or medically through manipulation of the hypothalamic-pituitary axis (luteinizing hormone-releasing hormone [LHRH] agonist/antagonist).[7]

While a patient is responding to ADT, PSA levels decline and stabilize and metastatic disease burden on imaging decreases in size. Patients in this disease state are considered to have hormone-sensitive prostate cancer. Unfortunately, the patient may experience an increasing PSA level and worsening of disease burden on imaging. Patients in this disease state are considered to have CRPC. CRPC is defined as having a total testosterone level of less than 50 ng/dL, with 2 consecutive rises in PSA with a PSA level of 2 ng/mL or more.[8] Generally, the average time it takes a patient with hormone-sensitive prostate cancer to develop CRPC is on average 2 years and thus these patients require close monitoring with physical examination, laboratory tests, and imaging.[1]

Over the last decade, advances in metastatic CRPC research have led to the development of several therapies designed to slow the progression of disease and improve the overall bone health of patients with CRPC. This article discusses relevant patient and treatment considerations in men with metastatic CRPC.

EVALUATION OF PATIENTS WITH METASTATIC CASTRATE-RESISTANT PROSTATE CANCER
General Considerations

History
The history in a patient with CRPC should include a discussion of urinary symptoms including, but not limited to, force of urine stream, urinary incontinence, hematuria, ability to empty, urinary frequency, and dysuria. Also, assess for weight loss, constipation, or bone pain. It is also important to evaluate neurologic symptoms such as fecal incontinence, saddle anesthesia, or numbness or tingling, because these can indicate signs of spinal cord compression, which requires urgent evaluation and management. Assessment of treatment-related specific side effects should be performed and are discussed later.

Physical examination
In addition to a standard physical examination, palpation of bony areas such as spinal column and hips may indicate bone metastases, which may require further evaluation and treatment.

Laboratory evaluation

Laboratory evaluation includes PSA, total testosterone, complete blood count (CBC), and comprehensive metabolic panel (CMP), specifically alkaline phosphatase for bony metastasis evaluation.

Imaging

Commonly used imaging modalities to evaluate the size, number, and character of metastatic lesions include bone scan, and cross-sectional imaging of the chest, abdomen, and pelvis with computed tomography or MRI. Dual energy x-ray absorptiometry (DEXA) is used to assess bone mineral density[7] (**Fig. 1**).

Frequency of visits

Patients with CRPC routinely undergo clinical evaluation every 3 to 6 months with laboratory and imaging tests based on the patient's clinical status.[7] In addition to assessment of disease status, visits focus on efforts to minimize treatment-related side effects and improvement of patient quality of life.

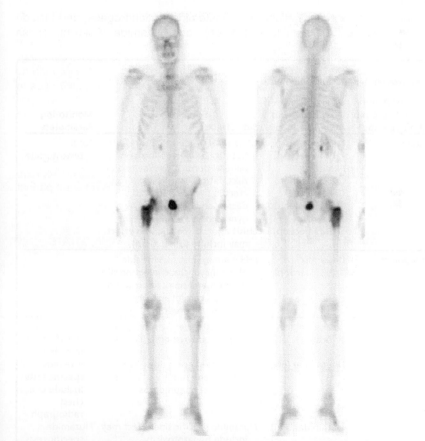

Fig. 1. Bone scan of a 48-year-old with metastatic CRPC. Findings demonstrated osteoblastic metastatic disease of the left scapula, lateral right seventh/eighth rib, right proximal femur, and left ischium. Nonspecific lateral L4 uptake, likely degenerative.

Adjunctive services

It is important throughout the course of CRPC to offer supportive services to patients. These supportive services can include pain management, social work, financial advisors, and nutrition. In addition to urologic evaluation, patients should maintain close monitoring with their primary care providers and cardiologists to provide comprehensive treatment and evaluation.[9]

TREATMENT CONSIDERATIONS
Androgen Deprivation Therapy

As discussed previously, patients with metastatic CRPC must continue lifelong ADT treatment. ADT can be accomplished through surgical castration (bilateral orchiectomy) or medically through manipulation of the hypothalamic-pituitary axis (LHRH agonist/antagonist) with or without antiandrogen (androgen receptor antagonist) therapy.[7] The advantages of surgical castration include rapid achievement of castrate levels of testosterone, cost-effectiveness, and benefits in patients who are poorly compliant (<50 ng/dL); however, the psychological impact of surgical castration must be considered in the counseling patients[10] (**Table 1**).

Oral therapy

The commonly used oral medications are nonsteroidal antiandrogens, and include bicalutamide (Casodex), nilutamide (Nilandron), and flutamide (Eulexin). These

Table 1
Medical androgen deprivation treatments

Mechanism of Action/ Category of Androgen Deprivation Therapy	Drug Name and Administration	Side Effects	Monitoring Parameters
LHRH agonist	Leuprolide (IM injection) Eligard (SC injection) Goserelin (SC injection) Triptorelin (IM injection)	General ADT side effects include hot flashes, decreasing bone mineral density, cardiovascular risks, fatigue and low energy, erectile dysfunction and decreased libido, gynecomastia, weight gain LHRH agonist specific side effect may include tumor flare	Total testosterone
LHRH antagonist	Degarelix (SC injection)	LHRH antagonist specific side effect may include injection site reaction and pain. Reported to have less cardiovascular risk than LHRH agonists	
Antiandrogen	Bicalutamide (oral)	Bicalutamide specific side effects may include dyspepsia, diarrhea	Bicalutamide specific tests include LFTs
	Nilutamide (oral)	Nilutamide specific side effect may include night vision loss, interstitial pneumonitis	Nilutamide specific tests include LFTs, chest radiograph
	Flutamide (oral)	Flutamide specific side effect may include hepatotoxicity	Flutamide specific tests include LFTs

Abbreviations: IM, intramuscular; LFT, liver function test; SC, subcutaneous.

medications block the binding of dihydrotestosterone (DHT) to the androgen receptor and thus translocation of the DHT–androgen receptor complex into the nuclei.[11] They are rarely used as primary ADT but are especially useful in prevention of a tumor flare when planning to start an LHRH agonist. In select cases, antiandrogen therapy is combined with an LHRH agonist. Such combinations are often referred to as combined androgen blockade and have shown conflicting results with regard to cancer outcomes.[12]

Ketoconazole (Nizoral) is an antifungal agent that is a potent inhibitor of both adrenal and testicular steroid biosynthesis and rapidly causes a decline in testosterone to castrate levels. Ketoconazole has been used to prevent a flare before starting an LHRH agonist and as a palliative option in patients with metastatic CRPC.[10] It is typically not used because of its toxic effects.[13,14]

Injection therapy

An LHRH agonist is a delivered injection that causes chemical castration. An example of this type of treatment is leuprolide (Lupron; Eligard). In the long term, it suppresses the pulsatile pituitary release of luteinizing hormone (LH), therefore decreasing the release of testosterone from the testes. However, on initiation of therapy there is an initial surge of testosterone, which may result in an increase in testosterone and potential increase in the burden of metastatic sites. This initial flare can cause significant morbidity, such as worsening pain and possible spinal cord compression. In order to prevent the flare from causing symptom increase or, in particular, spinal cord compression, patients are started on antiandrogen therapy for at least 2 weeks before undergoing LHRH agonist therapy.[11,15]

In efforts to prevent the flare associated with LHRH agonists, LHRH antagonists, such as degarelix (Firmagon) have been developed. Through competitive inhibition of the pituitary LHRH receptors, LHRH antagonists cause a reduction in the release of LH and thus decrease testosterone level without an initial flare.[15]

These LHRH agonist and antagonist injections can be delivered intramuscularly or subcutaneously at frequencies that range from every 1 month to every 6 months. In general, the side effects of ADT include hot flashes, decreasing bone mineral density, cardiovascular risks, fatigue and low energy, erectile dysfunction, decreased libido, gynecomastia, and weight gain.[16] There are specific treatment side effects as well, for example, nilutamide may cause night vision loss, injections are associated with injection site discomfort, and surgical castration causes body disfigurement and has surgical risks such as infection, anesthesia complications, and pain.

While on ADT, patients should maintain routine visits with primary care providers and their cardiologists. Efficacy of ADT is assessed through a total testosterone test to ensure a castrate-level testosterone, and, depending on which treatment is used, a CMP or simply liver function tests (LFTs) may be ordered as well.

Therapies for Castrate-Resistant Prostate Cancer

Sipuleucel-T

Sipuleucel-T (Provenge) is a form of immunotherapy and is often referred to as the prostate cancer vaccine. This treatment is indicated for asymptomatic or minimally symptomatic patients with metastatic CRPC and is typically given early in the treatment course.[17] The treatment consists of taking blood, then activating the mononuclear cells and fusing with a granulocyte-macrophage colony-stimulating factor to encourage T-cell proliferation.[17,18] The treatment starts with a blood collection process called leukapheresis, which takes about 3 to 4 hours and is followed 3 days later with a 60-minute infusion of sipuleucel-T (the patient's own immunostimulated blood cells). This therapeutic sequence is every other week for a total of 3 treatments (total of about 6 weeks). The patient is premedicated with acetaminophen and an antihistamine 30 minutes before the infusion.

The side effect profile of sipuleucel-T includes flulike symptoms, with the most commonly reported being back pain and chills. The symptoms typically last no more than 2 days. The patient is advised to eat a calcium-rich diet starting 2 to 3 days before leukapheresis.

The efficacy of sipuleucel-T is not assessed through laboratory work or imaging, because it does not generally create a quick change in disease status as shown by PSA monitoring or radiographic imaging. Overall it improves survival by 4 months (21.7 months vs 25.8 months in patients who received Provenge). The patients need a CBC and CMP before each therapy[12] (**Table 2**).

Enzalutamide

Enzalutamide (Xtandi) inhibits the androgen receptor and is used in men with metastatic CRPC before and after receiving chemotherapy.[19] It is a 40-mg capsule and it is recommended to take 4 capsules once daily. The most common side effects include fatigue, diarrhea, hypertension, and headache. It should be cautiously used in patients with history of neurologic conditions such as stroke and seizure. It can cause seizures, an increased rate of falls, and has been associated with posterior reversible encephalopathy syndrome (PRES), characterized by headache, confusion, and vision changes.[20] It has the convenience of having no required monitoring laboratory tests, although regularly scheduled appointments are recommended. Results from the AFFIRM study showed a survival benefit of 18.4 months in patients who received enzalutamide versus 13.6 months in those who did not.[21,22]

Abiraterone

Abiraterone acetate (Zytiga) is an androgen synthesis inhibitor through the blockade of enzymes 17α-hydroxylase and C17,20-lyase. It is a 250-mg tablet, and it is recommended to take 4 tablets once daily without food in combination with a low dose of oral prednisone. The addition of prednisone is to compensate for the decrease in cortisol and block the compensatory increase in adrenocorticotropic hormone.[23] Its side effect profile consists of fatigue, hypokalemia, hypertension, hepatotoxicity, nausea, vomiting, and diarrhea.[24] It should be used cautiously in patients with a history of cardiac disorder such as congestive heart failure. In addition to regular visits and checking vitals, patients need at minimum LFTs at least every 2 weeks for the initial 3 months, then monthly. In the COU-AA-302 study, abiraterone showed a survival benefit of 34.7 months versus 30.3 months for placebo.[25,26]

Radium-223

Radium-223 (Xofigo) is approved for men with CRPC and bony metastases, regardless of performance status. It is an alpha-emitting radioactive agent that targets and binds to areas of high bone turnover, as in metastatic bone lesions.[27] It is a coordinated effort, typically with radiation oncology, in which the patient receives an intravenous injection every 4 weeks for 6 injections. It is well tolerated with minimal side effects, including diarrhea, nausea, vomiting, and abnormal blood count, specifically in patients who have received chemotherapy prior to radium-223.[28] Radium-223 is reported to improve quality of life, survival, and median time to first symptomatic skeletal-related event (SRE). An SRE is defined as a pathologic fracture, spinal cord compression, need for radiation or surgery to the bone, or tumor-induced hypercalcemia. The overall survival benefit was 14.9 months in patients who received radium-223 versus 11.3 months in those who did not.[29]

Table 2
Castrate-resistant prostate cancer treatment options

Drug	Mechanism of Action	Regimen	Side Effects	Monitoring Parameters
Sipuleucel-T (Provenge)	Immunotherapy	250 mL IV q 2 wk	Flulike symptoms, specifically back pain, chills, headache	CMP, CBC
Enzalutamide (Xtandi) 40 mg	Inhibits androgen receptor and androgen receptor translocation	160 mg PO q HS	Seizure risk, PRES, hypertension, fatigue, nausea, vomiting, diarrhea, extremity edema	BP, routine tests, including CMP, CBC
Abiraterone (Zytiga) 250 mg	Inhibits androgen synthesis	1000 mg PO q HS (plus prednisone 5 mg PO BID), without food (no food should be eaten for at least 2 h before taking Zytiga or 1 h after)	Fatigue, hepatotoxicity, hypokalemia, hypertension, nausea, vomiting, diarrhea	Blood pressure, LFTs every 2 wk × 3 mo, then monthly
Docetaxel (Taxotere)	Microtubule inhibitor	75 mg/m^2 IV q 3 wk × 6 cycles (plus prednisone starting the day before infusion for a total of 3 d)	Nausea, vomiting, diarrhea, low blood counts, fatigue, infections, peripheral neuropathy, nail changes, hair loss	CMP, CBC with differential
Cabazitaxel (Jevtana)	Microtubule inhibitor	25 mg/m^2 IV q 3 wk (plus prednisone 5 mg PO BID)	Low blood counts, nausea, vomiting, diarrhea, fatigue, peripheral neuropathy, infections, hair loss, nail changes	CMP, CBC with differential
Radium-223 (Xofigo)	Alpha particle–emitting radioactive agent	IV injection q 4 wk × 6	Nausea, vomiting, diarrhea, low blood counts, peripheral edema, bone marrow suppression	CMP, CBC with differential

Abbreviations: BID, twice a day; HS, at bedtime; IV, intravenous; PO, by mouth; PRES, posterior reversible encephalopathy syndrome; q, every.

Docetaxel

Docetaxel (Taxotere) has been available for patients with metastatic CRPC since it was approved as first-line therapy in 2004.[30] Docetaxel causes apoptosis from inhibition of the microtubule assembly and is approved for use in patients with good performance status with or without symptoms. Docetaxel not only improved pain but also decreased risk of death. It is an infusion given every 3 weeks for 6 treatment cycles. It has many side effects, including low blood counts, fluid retention, peripheral neuropathy, nausea, diarrhea, hair loss, mouth sores, infection, and nail changes. To try to help prevent fluid retention and allergic reaction, prednisone is given at the time of infusion.[31] It has strict laboratory monitoring requirements with CMP and CBC with differential.[32]

Cabazitaxel

Cabazitaxel (Jevtana) is approved for patients with metastatic CRPC who have previously received docetaxel.[6] It is given through an intravenous infusion every 3 weeks in combination with prednisone. It has similar monitoring parameters and side effects as docetaxel.[33] It is recommended to combine cabazitaxel with a neutrophil growth factor supporting agent.[34,35]

ADJUVANT TREATMENT AND EVALUATION CONSIDERATIONS

The various therapies used to treat patients with CRPC have various treatment-related side effects that can cause morbidity and have negative effects on the quality of life of patients. Outlined here are various treatment strategies that can reduce treatment-related side effects.

Hot Flashes

A side effect of low testosterone, caused by ADT, can be hot flashes, which have the potential to be detrimental to the patient's quality of life. A 1-time intramuscular injection of medroxyprogesterone may help reduce hot flashes but has a side effect risk of deep vein thrombosis (DVT).[16] The daily oral medication megestrol acetate (Megace) may also benefit patients, although it also has the risk of DVT and weight gain.[16,36]

Gynecomastia

ADT may cause gynecomastia and, before starting therapy, the patients may undergo prophylactic radiation to the breasts for prevention.[37]

Bone Health

ADT causes demineralization of the bones, therefore leading to osteopenia and osteoporosis and an increased risk of SRE. An SRE is defined as pathologic fracture, need for radiation therapy or surgery to bone, or spinal cord compression.[38] It is recommended to get a baseline DEXA and repeat every 1 to 3 years based on risk. Standard recommendations include calcium 1200 mg and vitamin D 1000 IU daily and to continue weight-bearing exercise.[7,16] In addition, there are treatment options that have been shown to increase bone mineral density and decrease the incidence of vertebral fractures in men with prostate cancer. Denosumab, a RANK (receptor activator of nuclear factor kappa-B) ligand inhibitor that in turn inhibits osteoclastic activity within the bone, is indicated for use in men with and without bone metastasis.[39] Denosumab (Prolia) 60 mg is a subcutaneous injection given every 6 months for men without bony lesions in order to prevent osteoporosis, and denosumab (Xgeva) is 120 mg injected subcutaneously every month to prevent SREs. Side effects of denosumab include hypocalcemia and a CMP is needed before each injection.[38,40,41]

Zoledronic acid (Zometa) is also used for improving bone health by slowing the effect of osteoclasts on bone. Zometa is an intravenous infusion that has a side effect of flulike symptoms. It is also associated with a reduction in renal function.[42,43] Both therapies, zoledronic acid and denosumab, have the side effect of osteonecrosis of the jaw and it is recommended to have dental clearance before starting therapy.[41,43]

SUMMARY

Metastatic CRPC has many treatment options now, and more being developed. Although the best sequence of these treatments is yet to be fully determined, it is optimal to coordinate the therapies in a manner in which the patient receives full benefit from each individual therapy. It is wise to know the patient's goals, because this helps in developing the treatment pathway as well. Through a coordinated effort amongst the specialty practice and the general practitioner, a patient should have access to the customized care and treatment plan designed for him to improve survival and maximize his quality of life.

REFERENCES

1. Smith MR, Kabbinavar F, Saad F, et al. Natural history of rising serum prostate-specific antigen in men with castrate nonmetastatic prostate cancer. J Clin Oncol 2005;23(13):2918–25.
2. Cookson MS, Lowrance WT, Murad MH, et al. Castration-resistant prostate cancer: AUA guideline amendment. J Urol 2015;193(2):491–9.
3. Catalona WJ, Smith DS, Ratliff TL, et al. Measurement of prostate-specific antigen in serum as a screening test for prostate cancer. N Engl J Med 1991;324(17): 1156–61.
4. Siegel RL, Miller KD, Jemal A. Cancer statistics, 2017. CA Cancer J Clin 2017; 67(1):7–30.
5. Matsumoto K, Komatsuda A, Yanai Y, et al. Determining when to stop prostate specific antigen monitoring after radical prostatectomy: the role of ultrasensitive prostate specific antigen. J Urol 2017;197(3 Pt 1):655–61.
6. Pound CR, Partin AW, Eisenberger MA, et al. Natural history of progression after PSA elevation following radical prostatectomy. JAMA 1999;281(17):1591–7.
7. Mohler JL, Antonarakis ES, Armstrong AJ, et al. Prostate Cancer, version 2.2017 2017. Pros-B - Pros-G]. Available at: https://www.nccn.org/professionals/ physician_gls/pdf/prostate.pdf.
8. Harris WP, Mostaghel EA, Nelson PS, et al. Androgen deprivation therapy: progress in understanding mechanisms of resistance and optimizing androgen depletion. Nat Clin Pract Urol 2009;6(2):76–85.
9. Stratton KS, Moeller AM, Cookson MS. Implementation of the AUA's CRPC guidelines into practice: establishing a multidisciplinary clinic. Urol Pract 2016;3(3): 203–9.
10. Pokuri VK, Nourkeyhani H, Betsy B, et al. Strategies to circumvent testosterone surge and disease flare in advanced prostate cancer: emerging treatment paradigms. J Natl Compr Canc Netw 2015;13(7):e49–55.
11. Crawford ED. Hormonal therapy of prostatic carcinoma. Defining the challenge. Cancer 1990;66(5 Suppl):1035–8.
12. Schulze H, Senge T. Influence of different types of antiandrogens on luteinizing hormone-releasing hormone analogue-induced testosterone surge in patients with metastatic carcinoma of the prostate. J Urol 1990;144(4):934–41.
13. Food and Drug Administration. Ketoconazole label information. 2013. Available at: https://www.accessdata.fda.gov/drugsatfda_docs/label/2013/018533s040lbl. pdf.
14. Basch E, Loblaw DA, Oliver TK, et al. Systemic therapy in men with metastatic castration-resistant prostate cancer: American Society of Clinical Oncology and Cancer Care Ontario clinical practice guideline. J Clin Oncol 2014;32(30): 3436–48.

15. Schally AV, Block NL, Rick FG. Discovery of LHRH and development of LHRH analogs for prostate cancer treatment. Prostate 2017;77(9):1036–54.

16. Guise TA, Oefelein MG, Eastham JA, et al. Estrogenic side effects of androgen deprivation therapy. Rev Urol 2007;9(4):163–80.

17. Kantoff PW, Higano CS, Shore ND, et al. Sipuleucel-T immunotherapy for castration-resistant prostate cancer. N Engl J Med 2010;363(5):411–22.

18. Small EJ, Schellhammer PF, Higano CS, et al. Placebo-controlled phase III trial of immunologic therapy with sipuleucel-T (APC8015) in patients with metastatic, asymptomatic hormone refractory prostate cancer. J Clin Oncol 2006;24(19): 3089–94.

19. Beer TM, Armstrong AJ, Rathkopf D, et al. Enzalutamide in men with chemotherapy-naive metastatic castration-resistant prostate cancer: extended analysis of the phase 3 PREVAIL study. Eur Urol 2017;71(2):151–4.

20. Food and Drug Administration. Enzalutamide label information. 2014. Available at: https://www.accessdata.fda.gov/drugsatfda_docs/label/2014/203415s003lbl. pdf.

21. Fizazi K, Scher HI, Miller K, et al. Effect of enzalutamide on time to first skeletal-related event, pain, and quality of life in men with castration-resistant prostate cancer: results from the randomised, phase 3 AFFIRM trial. Lancet Oncol 2014; 15(10):1147–56.

22. Penson DF, Armstrong AJ, Concepcion R, et al. Enzalutamide versus bicalutamide in castration-resistant prostate cancer: the STRIVE trial. J Clin Oncol 2016;34(18):2098–106.

23. Auchus RJ, Yu MK, Nguyen S, et al. Use of prednisone with abiraterone acetate in metastatic castration-resistant prostate cancer. Oncologist 2014;19(12):1231–40.

24. Food and Drug Administration. Abiraterone label information. 2013. Available at: https://www.accessdata.fda.gov/drugsatfda_docs/label/2013/202379s007lbl.pdf.

25. Fizazi K, Scher HI, Molina A, et al. Abiraterone acetate for treatment of metastatic castration-resistant prostate cancer: final overall survival analysis of the COU-AA-301 randomised, double-blind, placebo-controlled phase 3 study. Lancet Oncol 2012;13(10):983–92.

26. Ryan CJ, Smith MR, Fizazi K, et al. Abiraterone acetate plus prednisone versus placebo plus prednisone in chemotherapy-naive men with metastatic castration-resistant prostate cancer (COU-AA-302): final overall survival analysis of a randomised, double-blind, placebo-controlled phase 3 study. Lancet Oncol 2015;16(2):152–60.

27. Parker C, Nilsson S, Heinrich D, et al. Alpha emitter radium-223 and survival in metastatic prostate cancer. N Engl J Med 2013;369(3):213–23.

28. Food and Drug Administration. Radium-223 label information. 2013. Available at: https://www.accessdata.fda.gov/drugsatfda_docs/label/2013/203971lbl.pdf.

29. Hoskin P, Sartor O, O'Sullivan JM, et al. Efficacy and safety of radium-223 dichloride in patients with castration-resistant prostate cancer and symptomatic bone metastases, with or without previous docetaxel use: a prespecified subgroup analysis from the randomised, double-blind, phase 3 ALSYMPCA trial. Lancet Oncol 2014;15(12):1397–406.

30. Tannock IF, de Wit R, Berry WR, et al. Docetaxel plus prednisone or mitoxantrone plus prednisone for advanced prostate cancer. N Engl J Med 2004;351(15): 1502–12.

31. Food and Drug Administration. Docetaxel label information. 2012. Available at: https://www.accessdata.fda.gov/drugsatfda_docs/label/2012/201525s002lbl.pdf.

32. Kellokumpu-Lehtinen PL, Harmenberg U, Joensuu T, et al. 2-Weekly versus 3-weekly docetaxel to treat castration-resistant advanced prostate cancer: a randomised, phase 3 trial. Lancet Oncol 2013;14(2):117–24.
33. Food and Drug Administration. Cabazitaxel label information. 2010. Available at: https://www.accessdata.fda.gov/drugsatfda_docs/label/2010/201023lbl.pdf.
34. de Bono JS, Oudard S, Ozguroglu M, et al. Prednisone plus cabazitaxel or mitoxantrone for metastatic castration-resistant prostate cancer progressing after docetaxel treatment: a randomised open-label trial. Lancet 2010;376(9747): 1147–54.
35. Di Lorenzo G, D'Aniello C, Buonerba C, et al. Peg-filgrastim and cabazitaxel in prostate cancer patients. Anticancer Drugs 2013;24(1):84–9.
36. Loprinzi CL, Michalak JC, Quella SK, et al. Megestrol acetate for the prevention of hot flashes. N Engl J Med 1994;331(6):347–52.
37. Gagnon JD, Moss WT, Stevens KR. Pre-estrogen breast irradiation for patients with carcinoma of the prostate: a critical review. J Urol 1979;121(2):182–4.
38. Fizazi K, Carducci M, Smith M, et al. Denosumab versus zoledronic acid for treatment of bone metastases in men with castration-resistant prostate cancer: a randomised, double-blind study. Lancet 2011;377(9768):813–22.
39. Smith MR, Saad F, Coleman R, et al. Denosumab and bone-metastasis-free survival in men with castration-resistant prostate cancer: results of a phase 3, randomised, placebo-controlled trial. Lancet 2012;379(9810):39–46.
40. Food and Drug Administration. Prolia label information. 2011. Available at: https://www.accessdata.fda.gov/drugsatfda_docs/label/2011/125320s5s6lbl.pdf.
41. Food and Drug Administration. Xgeva label information. 2010. Available at: https://www.accessdata.fda.gov/drugsatfda_docs/label/2010/125320s007lbl.pdf.
42. Conte P, Guarneri V. Safety of intravenous and oral bisphosphonates and compliance with dosing regimens. Oncologist 2004;9(Suppl 4):28–37.
43. Food and Drug Administration. Zometa label information. 2014. Available at: https://www.accessdata.fda.gov/drugsatfda_docs/label/2014/021223s028lbl.pdf.

Evaluation and Workup of Hematuria in Adults

Priyanka Tilak, PhD[a], Zain Z. Hyder, BS[b], Abby Moeller, PA-C[a],
Todd J. Doran, EdD, PA-C[c], Sanjay G. Patel, MD[a],*

KEYWORDS

- Adults • Microscopic hematuria • Gross hematuria • Guidelines • Evaluation
- Best practice

KEY POINTS

- Hematuria is the presence of blood in the urine and can be stratified into glomerular or nonglomerular causes as well as microscopic or gross hematuria.
- Nonglomerular hematuria can represent urologic disease ranging from infection to trauma to malignancy and requires further workup by a urologist.
- The use of laboratory and imaging testing is necessary to discern the cause of hematuria especially in those with high risk for malignancy.
- Triple-phase computed tomography urography is the gold standard in initially visualizing the urinary tract for stones or other lesions in the upper and lower urinary tract.
- For asymptomatic microscopic hematuria, cystoscopy should be performed on all patients older than 35 years or those with risk factors for urothelial malignancy (ie, chemical exposure, smoking history).

DEFINITION

Hematuria is defined as the presence of an abnormal quantity of red blood cells (RBCs) in the urine. It is classified as follows:

- *Microscopic Hematuria*

    Microscopic hematuria is defined as ≥ 3 RBCs per high-power field ($\times 400$ magnification) in a single properly collected urine sample.[1]
- *Gross Hematuria*

    Gross hematuria is defined as blood in the urine visible by the naked eye. Patients often present to the emergency department or at the physician's office after

---

Conflict of Interest: None declared.
[a] Department of Urology, Stephenson Cancer Center, The University of Oklahoma Health Sciences Center, 800 Northeast 10th Street, Oklahoma City, OK 73104, USA; [b] The University of Oklahoma School of Medicine, Oklahoma City, OK 73104, USA; [c] Department of Family and Preventive Medicine, College of Medicine, 940 Stanton L. Young Boulevard, Suite 357, Oklahoma City, OK 73104, USA
* Corresponding author.
E-mail address: sanjay-patel@ouhsc.edu

such an episode. Gross hematuria must be differentiated from other causes of discolored urine.[2] Causes of abnormal urine color are shown in **Table 1**.[2]

EPIDEMIOLOGY

The incidence and prevalence of hematuria varies widely depending on age, gender, and the population screened. Britton and colleagues[3,4] reported the prevalence between 13% and 20% in men older than 60 years; however, according to Messing and colleagues,[5–7] microscopic hematuria (detected by urinary dipstick) was found in 10% to 21% of high-risk and asymptomatic men older than 50. The prevalence of microhematuria in adults ranges from 2.5% to 21.1%.[8] Thorough examination and evaluation of these patients is necessary, as 5% of patients with microscopic hematuria[9] and 20% to 40% of patients with gross hematuria are likely to have an underlying malignant condition.[10]

ETIOLOGY

Hematuria can represent underlying disease, the causes of which can be benign or malignant. Microscopic hematuria is further classified into glomerular (hematuria from the glomeruli suggesting intrinsic renal disease and is not discussed further being beyond the scope of this article) managed by nephrologists and nonglomerular (hematuria from nonglomerular sites, such as renal pelvis, ureter, and bladder, suggesting a urologic etiology) managed by urologists. Glomerular from nonglomerular causes can be distinguished by the color or urine, presence/absence of RBC casts, degree of proteinuria, and presence of clots (**Table 2**). The most commonly reported causes of hematuria may include urinary tract infections (UTIs), urinary tract stones, bladder and kidney tumors, urethritis, benign prostatic hyperplasia (BPH), and prostate cancer.

The following are some of the common causes of hematuria classified by symptom and location (**Table 3**):

- *Infection*: cystitis, tuberculosis, prostatitis, urethritis, schistosomiasis.
- *Malignancy*: renal carcinoma, Wilms tumor, carcinoma of the bladder, prostate cancer, urethral cancer, or endometrial cancer.

Table 1
Causes of abnormal urine color

Color	Foods	Drugs	Condition/Substances
Red/Brown	Beets, blackberries, rhubarb, fava beans, aloe	Laxatives (eg, Ex-Lax phenolphthalein), tranquilizers (eg, chlorpromazine, thioridazine, propofol)	Porphyrin (eg, lead, mercury poisoning), globins (eg, hemoglobin, myoglobin)
Orange	Carotene-containing foods (eg, carrots, winter squash)	Beta carotene supplements, vitamin B supplements, warfarin, rifampin, Pyridium	Urochrome (eg, dehydration)
Green/Blue	Asparagus	Amitriptyline, indomethacin, cimetidine, promethazine	
Black		Methyldopa	

Table 2		
Characteristics of glomerular and extraglomerular hematuria		
Indication	Nonglomerular	Glomerular
Color (if macroscopic)	Red or pink	Red, smoky brown, or "Coca-Cola"
Clots	May be present	Absent
Proteinuria	<500 mg/d	May be >500 mg/d
RBC morphology	Normal	Dysmorphic
RBC casts	Absent	May be present

- *Trauma*: renal tract trauma due to accidents, catheter, or foreign body; prolonged severe exercise; rapid emptying of an overdistended bladder (eg, after catheterization for acute retention).
- *Inflammation*: postirradiation.
- *Structural*: calculi (renal, bladder, ureteric), simple cysts, polycystic renal disease, BPH, congenital vascular anomalies.
- *Hematological*: sickle cell disease, coagulation disorders, anticoagulation therapy.
- *Surgery*: invasive procedures to the prostate or bladder.
- *Drugs*: analgesics, anticoagulants, sulfonamides, cyclophosphamide, nonsteroidal anti-inflammatory drugs (NSAIDs), oral contraceptives, penicillin (extended spectrum), quinine, vincristine.
- *Others*: genital bleeding, menstruation, excessive exercise, Münchausen syndrome, or fabricated or induced illness by caregivers.

PATIENT HISTORY

Given the wide differential diagnosis of microscopic and gross hematuria, a thorough history, review of systems, and physical examination are essential in the evaluation of a patient with hematuria. History should be directed at using a system-based approach in conjunction with a localization-based approach to determine the cause of the hematuria. Ruling out major mimics of hematuria (beeturia, menses, drugs, vigorous exercise, trauma, or recent urinary instrumentation) should be considered, as it can prevent further unnecessary laboratory and imaging evaluation.

Important questions to include when taking a history:

- Have you experienced fever or chills?
  - Fever and chills could indicate an underlying UTI resulting in hematuria
- Do you have urinary frequency or urgency?
  - Irritative voiding symptoms (frequency or urgency) can be a sign of UTI or bladder malignancy
- Is the hematuria associated with pain?
  - Painless hematuria is more concerning for malignancy, whereas painful hematuria is more suggestive of an infectious or inflammatory cause
- Do you have flank pain? Radiation to the groin?
  - Flank pain and radiation to the groin can be indicative of ureteral obstruction or urinary tract stones
- When during urination does the blood appear?
  - Initial hematuria, blood or clots at the beginning of the urine stream, is a symptom of urethral cause
  - Terminal hematuria suggest prostatic or bladder neck source

Table 3
Anatomic classification of causes of hematuria

Location	Organ Site	Tumor/Malignancy	Inflammation	Stones	Anatomic Abnormality	Other
Upper urinary tract	Kidney	Renal cell carcinoma, renal pelvis urothelial cell carcinoma, renal lymphoma, angiomyolipoma, oncocytoma	Nephropathy, pyelonephritis, renal abscess, renal tuberculosis	Renal stones	Polycystic kidney disease, medullary sponge kidney, hydronephrosis, arteriovenous malformation	Hypercalciuria, hyperuricosuria, renal trauma, papillary necrosis, sickle cell disease, renal infarction
	Ureter	Ureteral urothelial cell carcinoma		Ureteral stones	Ureteral stricture, fibroepithelial polyp	Ureteral polyp, ureter vascular/ileal fistula
Lower urinary tract	Bladder	Bladder urothelial carcinoma, bladder squamous cell carcinoma	Bacterial cystitis, tuberculous cystitis, radiation cystitis, *Schistosoma haematobium*	Bladder stones	Vesico-ureteral reflux, cystocele, bladder papilloma, trabeculated bladder	Bladder diverticulum, interstitial fistula. endometriosis
	Prostate	Prostate cancer	Prostatitis	Prostate stone	Benign prostatic hyperplasia	Prostatic trauma/ procedures
	Urethra/Penis	Urethral cancer; penile cancer	Urethritis		Urethral stricture, urethral diverticulum	

- o Blood equally dispersed throughout stream that does not clot signifies renal origin
- Is the hematuria cyclic in nature?
  - o This can be a symptom of endometriosis or other gynecologic sources
- Have you lost weight?
  - o Unintentional weight loss could signify underlying malignancy
- Are you training for a marathon, decathlon, or so forth?
  - o New or vigorous exercise can be a cause
- Have you recently been in any accidents?
  - o Blunt or penetrating trauma must be ruled out
- Have you traveled recently to regions in which schistosomiasis is endemic?
  - o Schistosomiasis is associated with squamous cell carcinoma of the bladder
- Do you experience dribbling, weak stream, intermittent stream during urination?
  - o These obstructive symptoms are associated with benign prostatic enlargement, but can often indicate urinary obstruction from bladder, prostate cancer, or urethral cancer

Medications

- Are you taking medications that may cause hematuria?
  - o Analgesics, anticoagulants, sulfonamides, cyclophosphamide, or NSAIDs can commonly cause hematuria

Past Medical History

- Bleeding disorder or anticoagulation
  - o Coagulopathies and arteriovenous malformations, history of nose bleeds, or hemoptysis are causes of hematuria
- Rule out infection (UTI):
  - o Chronic cystitis/pyelonephritis, perinephric abscess can lead to bleeding
- Prior chemotherapy or radiation
  - o Pelvic radiation and cyclophosphamide are associated with malignancy
- Urinary retention
  - o Chronic indwelling catheter is a risk factor for malignancy

Past Surgical History

- Recent instrumentation/surgery
  - o Catheter insertion/removal and so forth cause trauma and bleeding
  - o Urinary tract surgery can be complicated by fistula formation
  - o Chronic catheterization can increase the risk for squamous cell carcinoma of the bladder

Social History

- Are you a current or former smoker? Are you exposed to passive smoking at work or at home?
  - o Smoking is strongly linked to bladder cancer
- Work in a field with exposure to chemicals or dye?
  - o Chemical/dye exposure is a risk for genitourinary (GU) malignancy

Physical Examination

- Focused abdominal examination
  - o Flank pain: suggestive of stone or malignant obstruction of kidneys
  - o Flank mass: suggestive of renal malignancy

- ○ Suprapubic pain: suggestive of UTI
- ○ Suprapubic mass: suggestive of bladder malignancy
- ○ Evaluation for trauma (broken ribs, pelvic fracture, perineal/scrotal bruising)
- GU examination
- ○ Perineal pain: suggestive of prostatitis
- ○ Vaginal bleeding: possible cause of urine contamination

HEMATURIA WORKUP

After completing a thorough history and physical examination, patients without obvious mimics of hematuria require further evaluation. This must be performed in all patients with gross hematuria in the absence of infection, as well as in patients with microhematuria who are older than 35, or those with risk factors such as smoking, irritative voiding symptoms, exposure to schistosomiasis, or chemical exposure. Confirmation of microscopic hematuria should be performed using a properly collected urine specimen with a formal microscopic analysis with reporting of the number of RBCs per high-power field. All patients with irritative voiding symptoms (urinary urgency or frequency), dysuria, suprapubic pain/tenderness, or fevers, should undergo a urine culture to rule out UTI. Cytologic examination of cells in the urine should be done to evaluate for urothelial malignancy in all patients with gross hematuria, patients with microscopic hematuria and suspicion of bladder urinary malignancy, or microscopic hematuria with negative initial hematuria workup. An estimate of renal function should be obtained as part of the initial evaluation and may include blood urea nitrogen, creatinine, and calculated estimated glomerular filtration rate, because intrinsic renal disease can have consequences for renal-related risk during the radiographic evaluation.[1] Once laboratory tests have been performed, radiographic studies are required to further work up causes of hematuria. These consist of intravenous urography, computed tomography (CT) urography, magnetic resonance (MR) urography, noncontrast CT + retrograde pyelogram + renal ultrasound. Direct visualization of the bladder and urethra (lower urinary tract) is also achieved by imaging with cystoscopy, which is oftentimes performed in the clinic using a flexible fiberoptic cystoscope.

The workup of hematuria includes the following:

- Urine studies:
- ○ Urine culture (if symptomatic for UTI)
- ○ Urine cytology to evaluate for urothelial cell carcinoma
  - ▪ All patients with gross hematuria, patients with microscopic hematuria and suspicion of bladder urinary malignancy, or microscopic hematuria with negative initial hematuria workup
- Cross-sectional imaging of the abdomen and pelvis with delayed contrast imaging
- ○ CT urogram of the abdomen/pelvis preferred imaging modality
- ○ Allows for evaluation of the kidney and ureter (upper urinary tract)
- Cystoscopy
- ○ Allows for direct visual evaluation of the urethra and bladder (lower urinary tract)

Indicated cases of hematuria require prompt urologic referral for timely care and appropriate evaluation, as urologists are best able to interpret appropriate radiographic imaging and perform cystoscopy.

LABORATORY TESTING

- *Sample collection:* Appropriate and contamination-free sample collection steps
  - (lid of the sample collection vial to be covered as soon as collected to avoid oxidation).
- *Urinalysis*
  - *Dipstick analysis:* Dipstick analysis is the initial first-line test to diagnose hematuria. The sensitivity of a urine dipstick test for blood varies from 91% to 100%, and the specificity varies from 65% to 99%.[11] The test detects the peroxidase activity of RBCs; hence, hemoglobin and myoglobin can cause a false-positive result. Other causes of false-positive results may include dehydration, exercise, povidone iodine, and oxidizing agents, as well as semen in the urine causing a heme reaction.[12,13] Causes of false-negative results include vitamin C (a reducing agent) and air exposure.[12] Due to these false positives and negatives, as per the American Urologic Association (AUA) guidelines, microscopic examination should confirm the findings.
  - *Microscopic analysis:* Microscopic analysis is the *gold standard* tool to diagnose microscopic hematuria, not urine dipstick. Most providers will send out their microscopic evaluations to a laboratory; however, some providers will prepare and interpret their microscopic analyses in the clinic with a microscope. When performing urine microscopy, proper care should be taken in preparing the sample. A fresh sample of 10 to 15 mL should be centrifuged according to laboratory standards. The urine microscopic evaluation not only confirms hematuria but also helps differentiate glomerular from nonglomerular sources of bleeding. In nonglomerular hematuria, the RBCs tend to be homogeneous and normal in shape. Blood clots do not occur in glomerular hematuria because of the presence of urokinase and tissue-type plasminogen activators in the glomerular filtrate.[12] RBC casts are virtually pathognomonic for glomerular hematuria, because the matrix of the cast is Tamms-Horsfall protein, which is secreted by the distal tubule. There is also a possibility that urine dipstick may be more accurate than urine microscopy when the urine is very dilute and has a specific gravity of less than 1.007. In case of diluted urine, RBCs may lyse and not be visible, causing the urine microscopic examination to be falsely negative for hematuria.[14]
- *Urine culture:* It is prudent to obtain a urine culture in patients with hematuria, particularly from those with irritative voiding symptoms or a history of urinary tract infection.
- *Urine cytology:* Cytology helps in determining the presence of cancer cells in the urine. The sensitivity for checking voided urine for abnormal cells ranges from 66% to 79% and the specificity ranges from 95% to 100% in case of bladder cancer.[15–17] Due to lack of reliability in patients with microscopic hematuria, it is recommended to perform urine cytology in patients with suspicion of bladder urinary malignancy or with an initial negative hematuria workup. All patients with gross hematuria should undergo urine cytology evaluation.

IMAGING

There are various imaging modalities used in evaluation of hematuria that can be used to image the urinary tract. Generally, these imaging modalities allow for diagnosis of upper urinary tract (kidney and ureter) pathology, whereas lower urinary tract (bladder and urethra) pathology is diagnosed via direct visualization with cystoscopy.

Given its relatively high sensitivity and specificity, CT urography (CTU) is the preferred technique for evaluation of hematuria. CTU of the abdomen and pelvis consists of a noncontrasted CT (evaluation for renal/ureteral/bladder stones), a contrasted CT (evaluation for enhancing renal masses), and a delayed phase (evaluation for renal pelvis and ureteral masses). Many patients have an iodinated contrast allergy or renal insufficiency and cannot undergo contrasted imaging and thus MR urography or noncontracted CT scan + retrograde pyelogram + renal ultrasound should be considered.

- Radiographic testing
  - *Intravenous urography (IVU) (oldest method):* IVU (also known as intravenous pyelography or IVP) has been the traditional and oldest imaging technique for evaluating hematuria. However, IVU may miss smaller renal masses, with sensitivity of 21%, 52%, and 85% for masses smaller than 2 cm, 2 cm to 3 cm, and larger than 3 cm, respectively, when compared with contrast-enhanced CT.[18] IVU also cannot distinguish solid from cystic masses, requiring another imaging technique, such as ultrasound or CT, to further characterize the lesion.[16] Further, IVU has relatively low sensitivity of 52% to 59% for detecting urinary tract stones.[19] Hence IVU is rarely used in the present day setting due to the several limitations mentioned previously and increased availability of cross-sectional imaging.
  - *CT urography (replaced IVU):* CT of the kidneys and urinary tract is better than ultrasound in detecting stones in patients with hematuria[15] and it has the highest sensitivity of 94% to 98%.[19] CTU is typically performed in noncontrast/contrast/delayed stages. Noncontrast helical CT is excellent for detection of urinary stones and hydronephrosis. Contrast CTU has increasingly superseded IVU when a urologic cause for hematuria is suspected, as a result of its higher accuracy in detecting lesions in the renal parenchyma and the rest of the urinary tract.[20] It involves the injection of iodinated contrast media, with subsequent high resolution nephrogenic phase to evaluate renal parenchyma, pelvis and ureter for neoplastic lesions. This is followed by a delayed excretory phase to examine the lower tract including bladder and urethra for filling defects. Important limitations of CTU include radio-sensitive populations (eg, pregnant women), as well as patients with renal insufficiency or allergies to contrast media.[9]
- *MR urography:* For patients with relative or absolute contraindications to CTU, such as renal insufficiency, contrast allergy or pregnancy, cross-sectional imaging alternatives exist in the way of MR urography with/without gadolinium contrast. Although it is poor at detecting stones, its sensitivity for detecting renal lesions is greater than 90% and is an acceptable substitute.[1] Currently, the US Food and Drug Administration warns against the use of gadolinium-based contrast agents in patients with a glomerular filtration rate less than 30 mL per minute per 1.73 m^2 due to the risk of nephrogenic systemic fibrosis estimated to be 4%.[9]
  - Noncontrasted CT + Retrograde Pyelogram + Renal ultrasound:
    Delayed excretory cross-sectional abdominal and pelvic imaging is necessary to evaluate the upper urinary tract and exclude upper tract malignancies. If contraindications to MR exist, such as metal in the body, a

final alternative of noncontrasted CT with retrograde pyelogram and renal ultrasound can be used.

- *Endoscopic testing*
  - ○ Cystoscopy

    The accepted reference standard for examining the bladder and urethra in patients with hematuria is direct visualization with flexible or rigid cystoscopy.[21,22] Cystoscopy is recommended by the AUA guidelines in all patients at least 35 years of age with microhematuria and in all patients with gross hematuria. For patients younger than 35 with microhematuria, cystoscopy may be performed at the discretion of the clinician based on the presence of risk factors for malignancy.

    For all patients with microscopic hematuria, negative imaging, negative urine cytology, and low risk for malignancy, the AUA does recommend cystoscopy, due to its low morbidity and its unique ability to visualize the urinary tract.[1]

With this evaluation strategy, a cause for hematuria is identified in roughly 57% of patients with microhematuria and 92% of patients with gross hematuria.[1] Malignancy is identified in approximately 3% to 5% of patients presenting with microhematuria and 23% of patients presenting with gross hematuria.

FOLLOW-UP

Following an unrevealing workup for hematuria, a urinalysis with microscopic analysis should be checked annually for at least 2 years. Patients with persistent hematuria after a negative initial evaluation warrant repeat evaluation for 3 to 5 years, especially in those with risk factors for urologic malignancy.

Box 1
Recommendations (American Urologic Association guidelines)

1. The assessment of the patient with asymptomatic microhematuria should include a careful history, physical examination, and laboratory examination to rule out benign causes, such as infection, menstruation, vigorous exercise, medical renal disease, viral illness, trauma, or recent urologic procedures.

2. Once benign causes have been ruled out, the presence of asymptomatic microhematuria should prompt a urologic evaluation.

3. The presence of dysmorphic red blood cells, proteinuria, cellular casts, and/or renal insufficiency, or any other clinical indicator suspicious for renal parenchymal disease warrants concurrent nephrologic workup but does not preclude the need for urologic evaluation.

4. Microhematuria that occurs in patients who are taking anticoagulants requires urologic evaluation and nephrologic evaluation regardless of the type or level of anticoagulation therapy.

5. A cystoscopy should be performed on all patients who present with risk factors for urinary tract malignancies (eg, irritative voiding symptoms, current or past tobacco use, chemical exposures), regardless of age.

6. The initial evaluation for asymptomatic microhematuria (AMH) should include a radiologic evaluation. Multiphasic computed tomography (CT) urography (without and with intravenous contrast), including sufficient phases to evaluate the renal parenchyma to rule out a renal mass and an excretory phase to evaluate the urothelium of the upper tracts, is the imaging procedure of choice because it has the highest sensitivity and specificity for imaging the upper tracts.

7. For the urologic evaluation of AMH, a cystoscopy should be performed on all patients aged 35 years and older.

8. The use of urine cytology and urine markers (NMP22, BTA-stat, and UroVysion fluorescence in situ hybridization) is NOT recommended as a part of the routine evaluation of the patient with AMH.

9. For persistent AMH after negative urologic workup, yearly urinalyses should be conducted.

Data from Davis R, Jones JS, Barocas DA, et al. Diagnosis, evaluation and follow-up of asymptomatic microhematuria (AMH) in adults: AUA guideline. J Urol 2012;188:2473–81.

Guidelines for Workup for Microscopic Hematuria

Various associations. such as the AUA and the American Family Physician, have published peer-reviewed, evidence-based guidelines for hematuria.[1,9] These guidelines overall generally share a similar evaluation strategy with minor differences. For a summary flow chart of the AUA microscopic hematuria guidelines, see **Boxes 1** and **2**, **Fig. 1**.

Box 2
Clinical pearls/handy tips

- Even if a dipstick test for hematuria is positive, a key question is whether this truly represents blood in the urine versus free myoglobin or hemoglobin. Confirmation of positive dipstick test should be performed with a microscopic analysis of the urine.

- The combination of hematuria plus proteinuria suggests glomerular disease and prompts further evaluation by a nephrologist.

- Many food and drugs either cause hematuria or discolor the urine and should be considered in the evaluation of hematuria.

- Smoking, heavy analgesic use, age older than 35, chemical exposure, and chronic cystitis or indwelling foreign body increase urinary tract tumor risk.

- All patients with gross hematuria, microscopic hematuria in those older than 35, or with risk factors (smoking, irritative voiding symptoms, or chemical exposure) should undergo prompt hematuria workup by a urologist.

- Hematuria workup consists of the following:
  ○ Urine cytology
    ■ All patients with gross hematuria, patients with microscopic hematuria and suspicion of bladder urinary malignancy, or microscopic hematuria with negative initial hematuria workup.
  ○ CT urography (preferred)
  ○ Cystoscopy

- Before referral to a urologist, referring providers may obtain CT urography after an estimate of renal function and a urine culture to expedite evaluation.

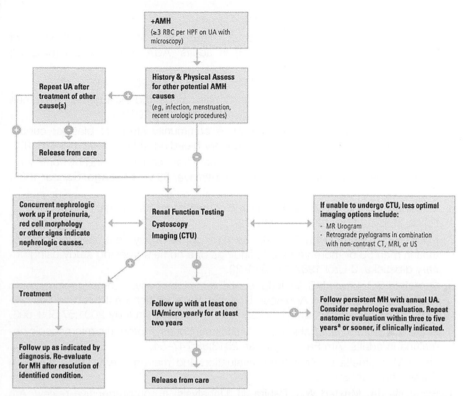

Fig. 1. Diagnosis, evaluation, and follow-up of AMH. [a] The threshold for reevaluation should take into account patient risk factors for urologic pathologic conditions such as malignancy. HPF, high-power field; MH, microhematuria; UA, urine analysis; US, ultrasound. (*From* Davis R, Jones JS, Barocas DA, et al. Diagnosis, evaluation and follow-up of asymptomatic microhematuria (AMH) in adults: AUA guideline. J Urol 2012;188:2473–81; and *Courtesy of* American Urological Association Education and Research, Inc, 2012.)

SUMMARY

The etiologies for gross and microscopic hematuria are vast and include multiple systems in numerous anatomic locations along the urinary tract. Organization of these etiologies using a combination of systems and anatomic approach can help the provider make the appropriate diagnosis and treatment. During the initial evaluation of the patient it is important to consider the mimics of hematuria to avoid unnecessary laboratory and imaging evaluation: typical foods such as beets and blackberries; drugs and supplements like NSAIDs, warfarin, and vitamin B; processes including dehydration, exercise and menses. Malignancy is a common cause of hematuria and it is paramount to identify risk factors such as a history of current or past tobacco use, chemical or dye exposure, or irritative voiding symptoms. Once mimics have been excluded and a diagnosis of gross hematuria or microscopic hematuria is established, it is imperative that one appropriately receive prompt evaluation by a urologist to work up hematuria with appropriate cross-sectional imaging, cystoscopy, and possible urine cytology.

REFERENCES

1. Davis R, Jones JS, Barocas DA, et al. Diagnosis, evaluation and follow-up of asymptomatic microhematuria (AMH) in adults: AUA guideline. J Urol 2012; 188:2473–81.
2. Sokolosky MC. Hematuria. Emerg Med Clin North Am 2001;19:621–32.
3. Britton JP, Dowell AC, Whelan P. Dipstick haematuria and bladder cancer in men over 60: results of a community study. BMJ 1989;299:1010–2.
4. Britton JP, Dowell A, Whelan P, et al. A community study of bladder cancer screening by the detection of occult urinary bleeding. J Urol 1992;148:788–90.
5. Messing EM, Young TB, Hunt VB, et al. Urinary tract cancers found by homescreening with hematuria dipsticks in healthy men over 50 years of age. Cancer 1989; 64:2361–7.
6. Messing E, Young T, Hunt V, et al. Home screening for hematuria: results of a multiclinic study. J Urol 1992;148:289–92.
7. Messing E, Young T, Hunt V, et al. The significance of asymptomatic microhematuria in men 50 or more years old: findings of a home screening study using urinary dipsticks. J Urol 1987;137:919–22.
8. Grossfeld GD, Litwin MS, Wolf JS, et al. Evaluation of asymptomatic microscopic hematuria in adults: the American Urological Association best practice policy—part I: definition, detection, prevalence, and etiology. Urology 2001;57:599–603.
9. Sharp VJ, Barnes KT, Erickson BA. Assessment of asymptomatic microscopic hematuria in adults. Am Fam Physician 2013;88:747–54.
10. Ismail M, Gomella L. Hematuria: evaluation and management. Urol Prim Care Physicians 1999;59.
11. Simerville JA, Maxted WC, Pahira JJ. Urinalysis: a comprehensive review. Am Fam Physician 2005;71:1153–62.
12. Ahmed Z, Lee J. Asymptomatic urinary abnormalities: hematuria and proteinuria. Med Clin North Am 1997;81:641–52.
13. Mazouz B, Almagor M. False-positive microhematuria in dipsticks urinalysis caused by the presence of semen in urine. Clin Biochem 2003;36:229–31.
14. Vaughan E, Wyker A. Effect of osmolality on the evaluation of microscopic hematuria. J Urol 1971;105:709–11.
15. Cohen RA, Brown RS. Microscopic hematuria. N Engl J Med 2003;348:2330–8.
16. Grossfeld GD, Litwin MS, Wolf JS, et al. Evaluation of asymptomatic microscopic hematuria in adults: the American Urological Association best practice policy—part II: patient evaluation, cytology, voided markers, imaging, cystoscopy, nephrology evaluation, and follow-up. Urology 2001;57:604–10.
17. Rodgers MA, Hempel S, Aho T, et al. Diagnostic tests used in the investigation of adult haematuria: a systematic review. BJU Int 2006;98:1154–60.
18. Warshauer DM, McCarthy SM, Street L, et al. Detection of renal masses: sensitivities and specificities of excretory urography/linear tomography, US, and CT. Radiology 1988;169:363–5.
19. Fielding JR, Silverman SG, Samuel S, et al. Unenhanced helical CT of ureteral stones: a replacement for excretory urography in planning treatment. AJR Am J Roentgenol 1998;171:1051–3.
20. Choyke PL. Radiologic evaluation of hematuria: guidelines from the American College of Radiology's appropriateness criteria. Am Fam Physician 2008;78: 347–52.

21. Rodgers M, Nixon J, Hempel S, et al. Diagnostic tests and algorithms used in the investigation of haematuria: systematic reviews and economic evaluation. Health Technol Assess 2006;10(18):iii–iv.
22. Stenzl A, Cowan NC, De Santis M, et al. The updated EAU guidelines on muscle-invasive and metastatic bladder cancer. Eur Urol 2009;55:815–25.

Kidney Stones

Brad Hornberger, MPAS, PA-C*,
Megan Rasmussen Bollner, MPAS, PA-C

KEYWORDS

- Kidney stones • Renal stones • Bladder stones • Nephrolithiasis
- Medical management • Surgical management

KEY POINTS

- Prevalence of kidney stones is increasing as more stones are found incidentally on CT and risk factors for stone disease (eg, obesity and type 2 diabetes mellitus) become more prevalent.
- Etiology of nephrolithiasis varies with stone type and depends on genetic, dietary, medication, lifestyle, and metabolic factors.
- Diagnostic evaluation of stone formers includes thorough history and physical, imaging, blood work, urinalysis, imaging, and analysis of stone fragments when possible.
- Medical and surgical management of stone disease includes increased hydration, dietary changes, pharmacological therapy for specific metabolic derangements, as well as, shock wave lithotripsy, ureteroscopy, percutaneous nephrolithotomy, and laparoscopic/robotic-assisted surgery.
- Nephrolithiasis during pregnancy requires special consideration in diagnosis, imaging, and treatment.

EPIDEMIOLOGY

Approximately 1 in 11 people in the United States is affected by kidney stones in their lifetime. The most recent data show prevalence in the United States of 8.8% for the period of 2007 to 2010, according to the National Health and Nutrition Examination Survey database. This represents an increase from 5.2% in 1988 to 1994 and 3.8% prevalence in 1976 to 1980.[1] A trend of increasing stone disease prevalence has been noted worldwide, although it is possible that this is partially attributable to incidental finding of asymptomatic calculi on high-quality CT scans.[2,3] Rates of stone disease vary with gender, race, age, comorbidities, and geography.

Disclosure Statement: The authors have nothing to disclose.
Urology, UT Southwestern Medical Center, 5323 Harry Hines Boulevard, Dallas, TX 75390-9164, USA
* Corresponding author.
E-mail address: brad.hornberger@utsouthwestern.edu

Physician Assist Clin 3 (2018) 37–54
http://dx.doi.org/10.1016/j.cpha.2017.08.006
2405-7991/18/© 2017 Elsevier Inc. All rights reserved.

Demographics

The prevalence of kidney stones peaks between ages 40 and 70 for men and between ages 50 and 60 for women.[2] Stone disease is more prevalent among non-Hispanic white men and women than other races and ethnicities. Urinary calculi are less than half as prevalent among black men as white men, and prevalence among Asian women is 45% lower than among white women.[4] Historically, white men have been more frequently treated for stone disease than white women (male-to-female ratio of 1.7:1), but recent data show that the gap between men and women is narrowing and is now closer to 1.3:1.[5] The same pattern is not seen among blacks and Hispanics, where women comprise 68% and 60% of stone formers, respectively.[6,7]

Environment

Because warm climates are more conducive to stone disease, calculi prevalence increases in the United States from north to south and from west to east, with the greatest prevalence in the southeastern United States.[8] Accordingly, the warm summer months have the highest incidence of stone disease and workers who are regularly exposed to extreme heat (such as steel workers) have higher rates of stone disease than those who work at room temperature.[9,10]

Comorbidities

Comorbid health conditions influence the likelihood that a person will form urinary calculi. Risk of stone disease rises with increasing body mass index, particularly in women.[11] For each element of metabolic syndrome (centripetal obesity, hypertension, elevated blood sugar, high serum triglycerides, and low high-density lipoprotein level) a patient has, the risk of stone disease increases.[12] The mechanism for the increased risk is not yet completely understood. It is possible that the low urine pH and increased excretion of urinary oxalate, uric acid, sodium, and phosphorus associated with obesity and insulin resistance could predispose stone formation.[13]

PATHOPHYSIOLOGY

The development of stones in the urinary tract has many etiologies. Diet, medication, lifestyle, genetic and metabolic variations all influence stone formation. The underlying pathophysiologic basis of stone formation is unique to each stone type and can be an indicator of an underlying disease. The metabolism of minerals, such as calcium, phosphorus, magnesium, and oxalate, all play a role in the progression or inhibition of kidney stone formation (**Table 1**).

Calcium-based stones are the most common, accounting for approximately 80% of all stones. Calcium oxalate is the most common stone type, making up approximately 60% of all stones. Calcium phosphate (brushite and apatite) stones account for 20% of stones. The remaining stones are uric acid, struvite, cystine, ammonium acid urate, and medication related (eg, triamterene and indinavir).

Calcium Stones

The formation of calcium stones is mediated through several factors. Supersaturation of calcium and oxalate in the urine promotes stone formation, as do several metabolic derangements, including low urine volume, low or high urine pH, high urinary excretion of calcium, oxalate, and uric acid, and low urinary excretion of citrate.[14]

Hypercalciuria

Hypercalciuria is the most common abnormality identified in calcium stone formers. Hypercalciuria is defined as greater than 300 mg/d for men and greater than 250 mg/d for women. The causes of hypercalciuria are excess absorption, excess resorption, and renal leak. *Absorptive hypercalciuria* is caused by excessive urinary calcium excretion due to excessive gastrointestinal (GI) absorption after a dietary calcium load. This is seen in approximately 30% of stone formers. Impaired renal tubular resorption of calcium leads to the development of *renal leak hypercalciuria*. This urinary loss of calcium drives the development of secondary hyperparathyroidism and increased vitamin D synthesis leading to increased bone resorption. This, in addition to increased GI absorption of calcium, leads to normal serum calcium levels. *Resorptive hypercalciuria* is associated with primary hyperparathyroidism, immobilization, and metastatic tumors. The excessive parathyroid hormone secretion in primary hyperparathyroidism leads to bone resorption, increased production of vitamin D, and increased GI absorption of calcium. This in turn leads to the development of increased urinary and serum calcium levels. Granulomatous diseases, like sarcoidosis, can also cause hypercalcemia and hypercalciuria.

Table 1
Types of kidney stones, prevalence, and risk factors

Type of Stone	Prevalence	Risk Factors
Calcium	75%–80%	Hypercalciuria Hyperoxaluria Hyperuricosuria Hypocitraturia Hypomagnesiuria
Uric Acid	8%–10%	Low urine pH Low urine volume Hyperuricosuria
Struvite/infection	5%–15%	Elderly Women Diabetics Urinary diversions Neurologic disorders Urinary stasis
Cystine	<1%	Inherited defect in renal transport of amino acids
Miscellaneous	1%	Laxative abuse Inherited disorder Excessive consumption of specific medications

Hyperoxaluria

Hyperoxaluria is another metabolic abnormality complicit in the formation of calcium oxalate kidney stones. Causes include primary hyperoxaluria, enteric hyperoxaluria, and dietary intake. Primary hyperoxaluria is a rare genetic condition with specific metabolic defects. Enteric malabsorptive states, including inflammatory bowel disease, celiac sprue, and intestinal resection, lead to the development of enteric hyperoxaluria. Diets rich in oxalate have been implicated in the dietary hyperoxaluria. Foods commonly identified as having high oxalate levels include nuts, brewed tea, potatoes, chocolate, and spinach.

Hyperuricosuria

Hyperuricosuria is defined as greater than 600 mg/d of urinary uric acid. It is caused most commonly by myeloproliferative states and excessive purine intake. It has been implicated in 10% to 40% of calcium stone formers.[15]

Hypocitraturia

Hypocitraturia is seen in 20% to 60% of patients with kidney stones evaluated metabolically.[16] Citrate inhibits kidney stone formation by binding to calcium and increasing its solubility. Although the most common cause of hypocitraturia is unknown, acid-base disorders and medications have been implicated.[17–19]

Hypomagnesiuria

Hypomagnesiuria is a known risk factor for formation of calcium stones. Magnesium binds to oxalate and reduces the urinary saturation of calcium oxalate. Low magnesium is also associated with low urinary citrate.[14]

Uric Acid Stones

Uric acid kidney stones account for up to 10% of all kidney stones.[20] Urinary pH drives the solubility of uric acid. As the urinary pH decreases so does the solubility of uric acid. In addition to low urinary pH, low urine volume and hyperuricosuria drive uric acid stone formation. In addition, recent findings point to the importance of insulin resistance in the development of uric acid kidney stones. Uric acid stones are seen in diabetic patients at a much higher rate than in the general stone-forming population. Low urinary pH is also seen at higher rates in patients with high body mass index and peripheral insulin resistance.[20,21]

Low urine pH

Low urine pH in uric acid stone formers likely has many contributing factors. Some investigators, however, have proposed a link between a reduction of excretion of ammonium in uric acid stone formers and insulin resistance.[22]

Low urine volume

Low urine volume has also been implicated in uric acid stone formation in workers exposed to high temperatures and living in warmer climates.[23,24]

Hyperuricosuria

As previously discussed, dietary factors play an important role in the development of hyperuricosuria.

Struvite/Infection Stones

Recurrent urinary infections by urease-positive bacteria (*Klebsiella*, *Pseudomonas*, *Staphylococcus saprophyticus*, *Proteus*, and *Ureaplasma urealyticum*) can cause struvite stones. These stones are composed of magnesium ammonium phosphate and are often implicated in staghorn kidney stones. Infectious stones account for 5% to 15% of all stones.[25] Patients at risk for struvite stones include the elderly, women, diabetics, and patients with urinary diversions, neurologic disorders, and urinary stasis.

Cystine Stones

An inherited defect in renal transport of amino acids has been implicated as the cause of cystine stones. With an incidence of 1 in 20,000, a high index of suspicion is required to identify patients. Factors that should increase suspicion include young age at presentation, family history, characteristic hexagonal cystine crystals, and mildly radio-opaque stones. In children, cystinuria causes up to 10% of all stones.[26]

The solubility of cystine is affected by cystine concentration, urine pH, ionic strength, and urinary macromolecules[13]; 24-hour urine collection shows urinary cystine excretion from 350 mg/d to 500 mg/d.[27]

Miscellaneous Stones

Xanthine stones are a rare stone type associated with an inherited disorder in the enzyme xanthine dehydrogenase or xanthine oxidase. Ammonium acid urate stones are associated with laxative abuse, recurrent urinary infections, recurrent uric acid stone formation, ileostomy, and inflammatory bowel disease.[28] Several medications have been implicated in inducing stone formation through various mechanisms. Promotion of calcium stone formation has been associated with loop diuretics and carbonic anhydrase inhibitors.[29] Medications, such as thiazide diuretics, corticosteroids, vitamin D, and antacids, can all indirectly promote stone formation. In addition, excessive consumption of medications, such as ephedrine, triamterene, sulfonamides, guaifenesin, silicate, indinavir, and ciprofloxacin, have caused stones composed of the drug itself.[29]

DIAGNOSIS

Assessing not only for conditions that affect the current stone event but also those that help predict the likelihood of future stone events is imperative.

Past Medical History

Assessing for a history of previous stone disease and family history of stone disease is an important part of the initial assessment. Chronic diarrhea, prior ileal resection, and inflammatory bowel disease are associated with risk factors that lead to development of uric acid and calcium based stones.[30] Patients should also be assessed for metabolic syndrome, gallstone disease, sarcoidosis, and previous bariatric surgery. Certain medications can increase risk of kidney stones. Assessing for active or previous use of medications, such as indinavir, carbonic anhydrase inhibitors, triamterene, loop diuretics, and dietary supplements, such as vitamin C and calcium supplements, is recommended.

Social and Dietary History

Not only can a patient's occupational history provide insight into the likelihood of chronic dehydration but also it can identify occupations in which early surgical intervention or more aggressive medical management is indicated. A dietary history is helpful to identify risk factors for stone formation and interventions to prevent recurrent stone disease. Knowing a patient's fluid, sodium, animal protein, and dietary oxalate intake is useful when discussing dietary interventions to prevent recurrent stones.

Physical Examination

A physical examination in patients with suspected nephrolithiasis is most useful to rule out other conditions. Colicky flank pain radiating to the ipsilateral abdomen or groin is a common presentation for an acute stone evident. Elevated blood pressure and tachycardia are often present. Elevated temperature could be an indication of an infected stone and requires prompt intervention. In addition, patients presenting with new-onset irritative voiding symptoms may be associated with a distal ureteral stone. Patients with a stable kidney stone disease are commonly asymptomatic.

Laboratory Evaluation

Basic metabolic panel and urinalysis are indicated in all stone formers. In patients presenting with an acute stone event or a fever, which could indicate an infected stone, a complete blood cell count with differential and urine culture should be considered. If borderline or elevated serum calcium levels are found, an intact parathyroid hormone to rule out hyperparathyroidism should be obtained. In addition, phosphorus and uric acid levels may be helpful. Acidic urine (pH <5.5) can be associated with uric acid stones, whereas more alkaline urine (pH between 6.5 and 7) is associated with the formation of calcium phosphate crystals. Renal tubular acidosis and infection with urease-producing bacteria are seen in higher urinary pH. Urine sediment should be examined for crystals. Hexagonal crystals are seen in cystinuria. Struvite stones are associated with rectangular coffin lid–shaped crystals. Tetrahedral envelope–shaped and hourglass-shaped crystals are described in calcium oxalate dehydrate and monohydrate, respectively.

Imaging

Abdominal x-ray films of the kidneys, ureters, and bladder (KUB); renal ultrasound; intravenous pyelogram (IVP); and noncontrast CT (NCCT) are commonly used imaging modalities to evaluate kidney stone formers. Radiographs are inexpensive and useful in imaging radiopaque stones large enough to be seen on plain film but have limited sensitivity and specificity. Ultrasound can assess for hydronephrosis and does not expose patients to radiation. The lower sensitivity of KUB and renal ultrasound, however, limits their usefulness compared with NCCT. A majority of patients with an acute stone event are evaluated with an NCCT, which has sensitivities and specificities of greater than 95%.[31] The Hounsfield units (HU) of a stone on NCCT can help predict stone type, which could have implications regarding treatment recommendations.

Metabolic Evaluation

Much debate surrounds which patients should undergo a metabolic evaluation for kidney stones. With first-time stone formers having a 50% risk of subsequent stone formation in 10 years,[32] selecting all patients to undergo a complete metabolic evaluation is not economically justifiable. Even in first-time stone formers, a discussion and shared decision making between patient and clinician should occur when deciding to pursue a metabolic evaluation.

First-time Stone Formers

Empiric fluid and dietary recommendations alone have been found to reduce rates of stone recurrence in first-time stone formers.[33] Although some studies have shown that first-time stone formers have the same incidence of metabolic abnormalities as recurrent stone formers,[34] a study by Yagisawa and colleagues[35] found that metabolic abnormalities are more common in recurrent stone formers. Even in first-time stone formers a thorough history and physical examination should be used to assess for underlying disease processes that may lead to recurrent stone disease and other complications. Patients with a family history of stone disease, urinary tract infections, gout, osteoporosis, and chronic diarrheal states have higher rates of recurrent stone disease.[36] In these patients, a thorough metabolic evaluation is recommended. In addition, all children presenting with stone disease and adults with cystine, uric acid, or struvite stones should undergo evaluation.

An abbreviated evaluation for first-time stone formers has been proposed (**Box 1**).[36]

Box 1
Abbreviated evaluation of single-stone formers

- History
  - Underlying predisposing conditions
  - Medications (calcium, vitamin C, vitamin D, acetazolamide, steroids)
  - Dietary excesses, inadequate fluid intake, excessive fluid loss

- Multichannel blood screen
  - Basic metabolic panel (sodium, potassium, chloride, carbon dioxide, blood urea nitrogen, creatinine)
  - Calcium
  - Intact parathyroid hormone
  - Uric acid

- Urine
  - Urinalysis
    - pH >7.5: suggestive of infection lithiasis
    - pH <5.5: suggestive of uric acid lithiasis
    - Sediment for crystalluria
  - Urine culture
    - Urea-splitting organisms: suggestive of infection lithiasis
  - Qualitative cystine

- Radiography
  - Radiopaque stones: calcium oxalate, calcium phosphate, magnesium ammonium phosphate (struvite), cystine
  - Radiolucent stones: uric acid, xanthine, triamterene
  - IVP: radiolucent stones, anatomic abnormalities

- Stone analysis

From Lipkin ME, Ferrandino MN, Preminger GM. Evaluation and medical management of urinary lithiasis. In: Wein A, editor. Campbell-walsh urology. 11th edition. Philadelphia: Elsevier; 2016. p. 1200–34.e7.

Twenty-four–Hour Urine Collection

Despite the added diagnostic and therapeutic information obtained by 24-hour urine collections, a minority of patients submit one for evaluation. A claims database of approximately 29,000 patients presenting with an acute stone event to an emergency department found that only 7.4% submitted a 24-hour urine collection within 6 months of the visit.[37] Controversy regarding the number of 24-hour urine collections needed and whether these collections should be completed while on a restricted diet exists. Some investigators recommend a baseline 24-hour urine collection and repeat testing after treatment recommendations have been made.[38] Urine creatinine can be used to assess the accuracy of the urine collection. Weight-based normal values for 24-hour urine creatinine are 15 mg/kg to 20 mg/kg for women and 20 mg/kg to 25 mg/kg for men. Urine collections that fall outside these ranges should be interpreted with caution.

MEDICAL TREATMENT

The goal of medical treatment of stone disease is to prevent recurrent formation. Conservative management and selective pharmacologic therapies are used to mitigate the urinary abnormalities known to encourage stone formation.

Conservative Management

Fluid management is a mainstay in dietary management of stone disease. The dilutional effect of and diuresis caused by increased fluid intake is thought to alter the supersaturation of stone promoters and prevent urinary stagnation.[39] Borghi and colleagues[40] showed that increasing fluid intake to achieve a urine volume of at least 2 L/day reduced recurrent stone formation by 45% compared with no active intervention. There is no high-level evidence supporting the benefit of one type of fluid intake over another; however, some evidence points to the protective benefits of carbonated water,[41] citric acid flavored soda,[42] and citrus juices (orange and lemon).[43,44]

Dietary alterations alone can reduce recurrent kidney stone formation in a significant number of patients. Dietary protein intake increases urinary calcium, oxalate, and uric acid excretion.[36] Protein restriction has been found to reduce urinary uric acid and increase urinary citrate in hypercalciuric patients.[45] A commonly suggested level of animal protein intake for stone formers is 6-8 oz/day or 1-2 servings. Investigators have found that the Dietary Approaches to Stop Hypertension (DASH) diet was associated with a lower risk of stone formation[46] and a higher DASH score was associated with a higher urinary citrate and an increased 24-hour urine collection volume.[47] Restricting sodium intake to 2000 mg/day is another commonly recommended dietary modification to prevent recurrent stone formation. High-sodium diets have been shown to increase urinary crystallization of calcium salts by influencing urinary calcium excretion and decreasing urinary citrate.[48]

The role of dietary and supplemental calcium intake in stone formation is complex. Current evidence suggests that patients should maintain a moderate calcium intake preferably from dietary sources. Dietary calcium restriction leads to an increased intestinal absorption of oxalate thus raising the overall supersaturation of calcium oxalate.[36] If patients require calcium supplementation, some investigators suggest that it should be timed with meals to help reduce urinary oxalate.[49] In addition, although supplementation with calcium citrate increases urinary calcium excretion, those effects are likely offset by the benefit of increasing urinary citrate excretion.

Avoiding dietary oxalate consumption is challenging because it is found in most vegetables. Recurrent stone formers with elevated urinary oxalate levels and underlying bowel abnormalities or those with a history of gastric bypass should consider a low oxalate diet.[50]

Pharmacologic Therapy

Although conservative recommendations of fluid management and dietary recommendations normalize urinary risk factors for stone formation in a significant number of patients, selective pharmacologic treatments should be initiated as indicated. Pharmacologic treatment strategies can be stratified by the abnormality identified during metabolic evaluation (**Fig. 1**).

Thiazide diuretics enhance renal calcium reabsorption, thus reducing urinary calcium excretion. A meta-analysis with a mean follow-up of 3 years showed a 47% relative risk reduction in stone recurrence rates with the use of thiazides.[51] Indapamide and chlorthalidone are thiazide-like diuretics that have been shown to reduce stone recurrence as well.[52,53] Treatment with thiazides is known to induce hypokalemia in 13% to 50% of patients. This hypokalemia can lead to hypocitraturia and potassium supplementation with potassium citrate is often advised.[54]

Allopurinol can be used to treat hyperuricosuria in patients unable to lower their urinary uric acid levels with a purine-restricted diet. It blocks the ability of xanthine oxidase to convert xanthine to uric acid.[55]

Potassium citrate has been shown to reduce stone recurrence rates in calcium stone formers by binding to calcium and thus decreasing the formation of calcium oxalate.[56] It is also used to treat distal renal tubular acidosis by improving metabolic acidosis and hypokalemia. A liquid formulation should be considered in patients with enteric hyperoxaluria who have rapid GI transit times. Potassium citrate helps

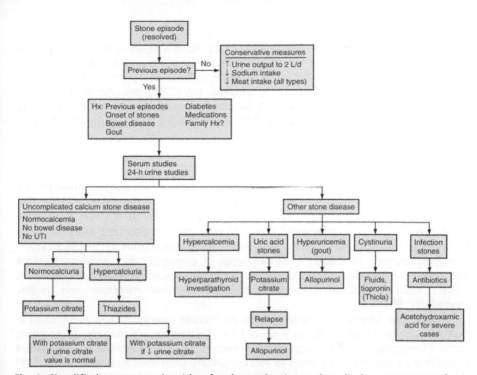

Fig. 1. Simplified treatment algorithm for the evaluation and medical management of urinary lithiasis. Hx, history; UTI, urinary tract infection. (*Adapted from* Lipkin ME, Ferrandino MN, Preminger GM. Evaluation and medical management of urinary lithiasis. In: Campbell-walsh urology. 11th edition. Philadelphia: Elsevier; 2016. p. 1200–34.e7.)

cystinurics and patients with uric acid stones by raising the urinary pH by providing an alkali load and increasing the solubility of cystine and uric acid. GI upset, abdominal pain, and diarrhea have been reported with use of potassium citrate.

Tiopronin use in kidney stone prevention is limited to cystine stones. Tiopronin is generally considered better tolerated than D-penicillamine and is the first-line drug in cystinurics. It contains a sulfhydryl group that is available to form a sulfide bond with cystine. Dosing of tiopronin is titrated to a dose that achieves urinary cystine levels of less than 250 mg/L urine (**Table 2**).

Table 2
Abbreviated list of most common medical therapy for recurrent kidney stone formers

	Typical Dosage	Most Common Side Effects
Hydrochlorothiazide	25 mg twice daily	Hypokalemia
Indapamide	2.5 mg daily	Hypocitraturia
Chlorthalidone	25–50 mg daily	Hyperuricosuria
Potassium citrate	20 mEq bid–tid	Hyperkalemia GI upset
Allopurinol	300 mg daily	Rash Myalgia
Tiopronin	800 mg divided doses tid; titrate dosage urinary cystine <250 mg/L	Dermatologic GI issues

SURGICAL MANAGEMENT

Technological advancements have driven kidney stone surgery toward less invasive techniques while maintaining high treatment success rates and lowering morbidity. The current armamentarium for surgical treatment of kidney and ureteral stones includes shock wave lithotripsy (SWL), ureteroscopy (URS), percutaneous nephrolithotomy (PCNL), and laparoscopic/robotic-assisted surgery. The most appropriate surgical treatment approach is dictated by stone-related factors, anatomic factors, and patient factors.

Renal Stones

Most asymptomatic nonstaghorn renal stones do not require surgical intervention. Patients with asymptomatic stones, however, have an approximate 50% risk of developing stone-related symptoms or stone growth at 5 years.[57] Overall, there is a 10% to 20% chance of a patient with an asymptomatic stone needing to undergo surgical intervention at 3 years to 4 years from initial discovery.[58] The management of staghorn stones, even if asymptomatic, involves a more aggressive approach. Untreated staghorn stones are associated with recurrent urinary tract infections, urosepsis, decline in renal function, and higher mortality.[59–62]

Preoperative laboratory evaluation should include urinalysis and urine culture. Culture specific antibiotic therapy should be initiated before surgery. In addition, some investigators have advocated for empiric antibiotics treatment 1 week before stone-related surgery in an effort to reduce urinary tract infections and sepsis.[63,64] Serum chemistries assess baseline renal function and provide insight into systemic diseases, which may predispose a patient to stone disease. If laparoscopic surgery, open stone surgery, or PCNL is performed, a baseline complete blood cell count is recommended. In kidneys with less than 15% function, nephrectomy should be considered.

The stone burden, location, and composition all play a role determining the most appropriate surgical technique for a patient requiring a stone-related procedure. If the composition of the stone is not known, HUs based on a preoperative NCCT scan can help guide decision making as well. The higher the HU, the more resistant a stone is to fragmentation by SWL. Treatment approaches are frequently grouped by overall stone burden less than 1 cm, between 1 cm and 2 cm, and greater than 2 cm.

For stones burden of less than 1 cm, SWL is a first-line treatment. With the diffusion of training and use of flexible URS, however, it is now considered an alternative first-line therapy. Stones located in the lower pole, those with higher HU, and those with a skin-to-stone distance of greater than 10 cm maybe be better treated with URS or PCNL. When assessed by post-treatment KUB or renal ultrasound, stone-free rates with SWL range from 50% to 90%.[58] In high-volume stone centers, URS has been shown to have stone-free rates of 80% to 100%.[65,66] PCNL is reserved for SWL and URS failures or in patients with unique anatomic issues.

For stone burden between 1 cm and 2 cm, the stone-related factors, discussed previously, and patient anatomic factors play an even more important role in choosing the proper treatment. Success rates of SWL and URS decrease and the likely need for PCNL increases with larger lower pole stone burden, increasing skin-to-stone distance, and unfavorable calyx anatomy. SWL is still the favored first-line approach in patients with favorable risk factors for success. When these factors are not present,

URS or PCNL is generally favored. Stone-free rates associated with SWL and URS vary based on the stone location. Reported success rates for SWL with upper pole stones (71.8%), middle (76.5%), and lower (37%) have been reported by Saw and Lingeman.[67] Single-treatment success rates with URS for stones between 1 cm and 2 cm is 90% in the upper and middle calyces and 80% in the lower pole calyces.[68] Stone-free rates with PCNL are independent of stone location and are greater than 90%.[69] The higher morbidity associated with PCNL has tempered its widespread use in stones less than 2 cm in size; however, it should be considered in lower pole stones greater than 1 cm in size.

Stone burdens greater than 2 cm should be primarily addressed by PCNL. Staged procedures should be considered if SWL and URS are attempted in stone burdens greater than 2 cm. PCNL has been shown to have stone-free rates of 95% in 1 series.[70] Poor success rates of less than 30% have been reported with SWL monotherapy in large stone burdens.[71] URS often requires staged procedures and has been shown to have a success rate of 75%.[72] Complication rates associated with PCNL from contemporary series have shown blood transfusion rates of 5% to 10% and 1% incidence of sepsis and delayed bleeding. In addition to lower stone-free rates and increased likelihood of the need of secondary procedures, SWL has been associated with a 23% incidence of steinstrasse (blockage of the ureter by stone fragments).[73]

Staghorn stones should be treated with PCNL and frequently require staged procedures. Poorly functioning or nonfunctioning kidneys and those associated with xanthogranulomatous pyelonephritis often require nephrectomy.

Finally, laparoscopic and robotic approaches are most commonly used in stone treatment during pyeloplasty to repair ureteropelvic junction obstruction where simultaneous pyelolithotomy or nephrolithotomy is an extension of the main surgical procedure. Although PCNL is generally considered first-line treatment of most calyceal diverticular stones, a laparoscopic or robotic approach could be considered for anteriorly located diverticular stones (**Box 2**).

Ureteral Stones

Surgical treatment of ureteral stones involves the same modalities used to treat renal stones. In addition to stone-related factors, clinical factors and technical factors all play a role in determining the optimum treatment modality.

Ureteral obstruction by a stone is mediated by the diameter and the location of the stone at presentation. For ureteral stones less than 5 mm is size, there is a 68% chance of spontaneous stone passage, whereas stones between 6 mm and 10 mm have a 47% chance of passage.[74] A review by Morese and Resnick[75] demonstrated a 22% chance of stone passage for stones presenting in the proximal ureter and 71% passage rate with distal ureteral stones.

Box 2
Risk factors for shock wave lithotripsy treatment failure
Lower pole stone
Stone with less than 900 HU on CT scan
Skin-to-stone distance greater than 10 cm
Larger stone burden
Unfavorable calyceal anatomy
History of SWL resistant stones (brushite, calcium oxalate monohydrate, cysteine)

Pharmacologic therapy has been used to enhance stone passage rates, reduce time to stone passage, and decrease analgesic requirements. Medical expulsive therapy with α-receptor blockers and calcium channel blockers have been the most studied, with α-blockers seeming to have the greater efficacy. α-Blockers have been shown to increase likelihood of spontaneous stone passage by 29% for all ureteral stones.[58] Higher rates have been reported with distal stones compared with proximal stones. A 50% improvement in distal ureteral stone passage has been reported with their role in proximal stones yet to be fully determined.[76]

The pretreatment assessment of patients with ureteral stones is similar to that of patients with renal stones; however, additional attention is required to the duration of symptoms and presence of acute renal injury. Also, a lower threshold for immediate intervention should be given to those patients presenting with fever. The presence of fever in a patient with a ureteral stone should be assumed to be related to urinary tract infection, whereas an elevated white blood cell count can be associated with physiologic stress or infection. Coagulation status, comorbid medical conditions, and body habitus should also be taken into account when deciding on a treatment modality.

As discussed previously, stone location plays an important role in treatment decision making. When stones are located in the proximal and midureter, the size of the stone is of utmost importance. Surgical intervention is more likely necessary for stones presenting in these locations because of the lower spontaneous stone passage rates and the questionable benefit of medical expulsive therapy, discussed previously. Patient preference, recurring severe pain, and failure of spontaneous stone passage in an approximate 4-week time period[77] are all indications for moving forward with treatment. Similar to renal stones, the additional factors that affect SWL success rates, including stone type, HU, and skin-to-stone distance, must be taken into account when considering treatment options. Success rates for SWL treatment of proximal and midureteral stones are 82% and 73%, respectively.[74] URS has been showed to have success rates comparable to SWL, at 81% for proximal and 86% for midureteral stones.[74] Generally, success rates for SWL and URS decline if stones are larger than 1 cm. In these cases, consideration for PCNL with an antegrade ureteroscopic approach could be considered.[78] Stones located in the distal ureter are more likely to spontaneously pass with a trial of stone passage. For those who do require intervention, SWL has a success rate of 86% and 74%, respectively, in stones less than 1 cm and greater than 1 cm.[74] URS success rates are slightly higher with 97% in stones less than 1 cm and 93% in stones greater than 1 cm.[74]

NEPHROLITHIASIS IN PREGNANCY

The rate of symptomatic kidney stones during pregnancy is low and is the same as the rate for nonpregnant women.[79–82] Patients usually present in the second trimester or third trimester with new-onset flank pain radiating to the groin or lower abdomen (90%), microscopic or gross hematuria (75–95%), and pyuria (40%) and are frequently misdiagnosed with appendicitis, diverticulitis, or placental abruption.[79]

Some physiologic changes of pregnancy increase the chances of stone formation: increased renal blood flow leads to increased glomerular filtration rate and thus increased calcium, sodium, and uric acid excretion; urine pH rises; and urinary stasis occurs secondary to increased progesterone and pressure from the gravid uterus on the ureters.[83] These lithogenic factors are mitigated by an increase in excretion of inhibitors, such as citrate, magnesium, and glycoproteins, so the rate of symptomatic stones is equal for pregnant and nonpregnant women of childbearing age.[55] Calcium phosphate stones are the most common in pregnancy.[84]

Diagnosis

Because the physiologic changes of the urinary tract are temporary, metabolic evaluation of pregnant stone formers is not generally performed until a patient has delivered and returned to the usual state of health.[36] When an obstructing stone is suspected in a pregnant patient, ultrasound is the first-line diagnostic modality because it avoids fetal radiation exposure and can diagnose secondary signs of obstruction, such as hydronephrosis and hydroureter, although some degree of hydronephrosis is a normal physiologic change in pregnancy. Color Doppler ultrasound can help distinguish the iliac vessels from a dilated ureter and identify ureteral jets of urine in the bladder. The unilateral absence of a ureteral jet is strongly indicative of obstruction.[85] If renal and pelvic ultrasound are nondiagnostic, transvaginal ultrasound sometimes identifies distal ureteral stones.[86] If all ultrasounds are negative, a trial of symptomatic treatment can be attempted by hydrating the patient and having her lie on her side with the symptomatic side up to relieve the pressure of the gravid uterus.[87,88]

If further diagnostics are needed after renal, pelvic, and transvaginal ultrasound and a trial of symptomatic therapy, magnetic resonance imaging without contrast, limited IVP (consisting of only 2 or 3 plates, 0.3–0.6 total rad), or low-dose CT (0.2–1.3 rad) may be used, with magnetic resonance or IVP preferred when possible.[89] Low-dose CT can be used in the second and third trimesters when organogenesis is complete.[90] The American College of Obstetricians and Gynecologists endorses the use of low-dose CT when clinically appropriate, because exposure to less than 5 rad is not associated with the development of fetal anomalies or fetal loss.[91]

Treatment

Although a majority (50%–85%) of stones in pregnant patients pass spontaneously, renal colic is still the most common nonobstetric cause for hospital admission while pregnant.[79,80] Symptomatic stones are not without significant morbidity: renal colic, infections, and urinary obstruction are all associated with premature labor.[92] While waiting for stone passage, acetaminophen is the safest pain medication in pregnancy. The α-blocker tamsulosin is a pregnancy category B medication and has been found in small studies of short-term use (3 days) to be safe for mother and fetus.[93]

For patients who are septic, have persistent severe pain, or have an obstructed solitary kidney, cystoscopy with ureteral stent insertion, URS, or placement of a nephrostomy tube is required.[83,94] The risk of stent encrustation is higher in pregnancy, and frequent stent exchanges (every 4–6 weeks until delivery) should be completed.[83] Stent placement and nephrostomy tube placement can temporarily relieve obstruction but necessitate a definitive procedure in the postpartum period to remove the offending stone. SWL and PCNL are not appropriate for use in the pregnant population.[95]

SUMMARY

Given the increasing prevalence of kidney stones and corresponding rising cost of treatment, it is imperative that clinicians are well versed in the diagnosis and management of nephrolithiasis. Advances in imaging techniques, medical management, and refinement in surgical interventions have improved the ability to diagnose and treat kidney stones, but chronic or prolific stone formers remain a clinical challenge. Continued advances in basic science, clinical research, medical management, and surgical intervention are necessary for the future of stone treatment.

REFERENCES

1. Scales CD, Smith AC, Hanley JM, et al. Prevalence of kidney stones in the United States. Eur Urol 2012;62(1):160–5.
2. Romero V, Akpinar H, Assimos DG. Kidney stones: a global picture of prevalence, incidence, and associated risk factors. Rev Urol 2010;12(2–3):e86–96.
3. Boyce CJ, Pickhardt PJ, Lawrence EM, et al. Prevalence of urolithiasis in asymptomatic adults: objective determination using low dose noncontrast computerized tomography. J Urol 2010;183(3):1017–21.
4. Soucie JM, Thun MJ, Coates RJ, et al. Demographic and geographic variability of kidney stones in the United States. Kidney Int 1994;46(3):893–9.
5. Scales CD, Curtis LH, Norris RD, et al. Changing gender prevalence of stone disease. J Urol 2007;177(3):979–82.
6. Sarmina I, Spirnak JP, Resnick MI. Urinary lithiasis in the black population: an epidemiological study and review of the literature. J Urol 1987;138(1):14–7.
7. Michaels EK, Nakagawa Y, Miura N, et al. Racial variation in gender frequency of calcium urolithiasis. J Urol 1994;152(6 Pt 2):2228–31.
8. Soucie JM, Coates RJ, McClellan W, et al. Relation between geographic variability in kidney stones prevalence and risk factors for stones. Am J Epidemiol 1996;143(5):487–95.
9. Prince CL, Scardino PL. A statistical analysis of ureteral calculi. J Urol 1960;83: 561–5.
10. Atan L, Andreoni C, Ortiz V, et al. High kidney stone risk in men working in steel industry at hot temperatures. Urology 2005;65(5):858–61.
11. Curhan GC, Willett WC, Rimm EB, et al. Body size and risk of kidney stones. J Am Soc Nephrol 1998;9(9):1645–52.
12. West B, Luke A, Durazo-Arvizu RA, et al. Metabolic syndrome and self-reported history of kidney stones: the National Health and Nutrition Examination Survey (NHANES III) 1988-1994. Am J Kidney Dis 2008;51(5):741–7.
13. Pearle MS, Antonelli JA, Lotan Y. Urinary lithiasis: etiology, epidemiology, and pathogenesis. In: Wein AJ, editor. Campbell-walsh urology. 11th edition. Amsterdam: Elsevier; 2016. p. 1170–99. Available at: https://www.clinicalkey.com/#!/content/book/3-s2.0-B9781455775675000510. Accessed April 27, 2017.
14. Park S, Pearle MS. Pathophysiology and management of calcium stones. Urol Clin North Am 2007;34(3):323–34.
15. Preminger GM. Renal calculi: pathogenesis, diagnosis, and medical therapy. Semin Nephrol 1992;12(2):200–16.
16. Zuckerman JM, Assimos DG. Hypocitraturia: pathophysiology and medical management. Rev Urol 2009;11(3):134–44.
17. Hamm LL, Hering-Smith KS. Pathophysiology of hypocitraturic nephrolithiasis. Endocrinol Metab Clin North Am 2002;31(4):885–93, viii.
18. Welch BJ, Graybeal D, Moe OW, et al. Biochemical and stone-risk profiles with topiramate treatment. Am J Kidney Dis 2006;48(4):555–63.
19. Melnick JZ, Preisig PA, Haynes S, et al. Converting enzyme inhibition causes hypocitraturia independent of acidosis or hypokalemia. Kidney Int 1998;54(5): 1670–4.

20. Maalouf NM, Cameron MA, Moe OW, et al. Novel insights into the pathogenesis of uric acid nephrolithiasis. Curr Opin Nephrol Hypertens 2004;13(2):181–9.
21. Abate N, Chandalia M, Cabo-Chan AV, et al. The metabolic syndrome and uric acid nephrolithiasis: novel features of renal manifestation of insulin resistance. Kidney Int 2004;65(2):386–92.
22. Sakhaee K, Adams-Huet B, Moe OW, et al. Pathophysiologic basis for normouricosuric uric acid nephrolithiasis. Kidney Int 2002;62(3):971–9.
23. Borghi L, Meschi T, Amato F, et al. Hot occupation and nephrolithiasis. J Urol 1993;150(6):1757–60.
24. Shekarriz B, Stoller ML. Uric acid nephrolithiasis: current concepts and controversies. J Urol 2002;168(4 Pt 1):1307–14.
25. Levy FL, Adams-Huet B, Pak CY. Ambulatory evaluation of nephrolithiasis: an update of a 1980 protocol. Am J Med 1995;98(1):50–9.
26. Knoll T, Zöllner A, Wendt-Nordahl G, et al. Cystinuria in childhood and adolescence: recommendations for diagnosis, treatment, and follow-up. Pediatr Nephrol 2005;20(1):19–24.
27. Coe FL, Evan A, Worcester E. Kidney stone disease. J Clin Invest 2005;115(10):2598–608.
28. Soble JJ, Hamilton BD, Streem SB. Ammonium acid urate calculi: a reevaluation of risk factors. J Urol 1999;161(3):869–73.
29. Matlaga BR, Shah OD, Assimos DG. Drug-induced urinary calculi. Rev Urol 2003;5(4):227–31.
30. Finkielstein VA, Goldfarb DS. Strategies for preventing calcium oxalate stones. CMAJ 2006;174(10):1407–9.
31. Chen MY, Zagoria RJ, Saunders HS, et al. Trends in the use of unenhanced helical CT for acute urinary colic. AJR Am J Roentgenol 1999;173(6):1447–50.
32. Uribarri J, Oh MS, Carroll HJ. The first kidney stone. Ann Intern Med 1989;111(12):1006–9.
33. Borghi L, Meschi T, Amato F, et al. Urinary volume, water and recurrences in idiopathic calcium nephrolithiasis: a 5-year randomized prospective study. J Urol 1996;155(3):839–43.
34. Pak CY. Should patients with single renal stone occurrence undergo diagnostic evaluation? J Urol 1982;127(5):855–8.
35. Yagisawa T, Chandhoke PS, Fan J. Metabolic risk factors in patients with first-time and recurrent stone formations as determined by comprehensive metabolic evaluation. Urology 1998;52(5):750–5.
36. Lipkin ME, Ferrandino MN, Preminger GM. Evaluation and medical management of urinary lithiasis. In: Wein A, editor. Campbell-walsh urology. 11th edition. Philadelphia: Elsevier; 2016. p. 1200–34.e7. Available at: https://www.clinicalkey.com/#!/content/book/3-s2.0-B9781455775675000522. Accessed April 29, 2017.
37. Milose JC, Kaufman SR, Hollenbeck BK, et al. Prevalence of 24-hour urine collection in high risk stone formers. J Urol 2014;191(2):376–80.
38. Goldfarb DS, Arowojolu O. Metabolic evaluation of first-time and recurrent stone formers. Urol Clin North Am 2013;40(1):13–20.
39. Pak CY, Sakhaee K, Crowther C, et al. Evidence justifying a high fluid intake in treatment of nephrolithiasis. Ann Intern Med 1980;93(1):36–9.
40. Borghi L, Meschi T, Schianchi T, et al. Urine volume: stone risk factor and preventive measure. Nephron 1999;81(Suppl 1):31–7.
41. Coen G, Sardella D, Barbera G, et al. Urinary composition and lithogenic risk in normal subjects following oligomineral versus bicarbonate-alkaline high calcium mineral water intake. Urol Int 2001;67(1):49–53.

42. Haleblian GE, Leitao VA, Pierre SA, et al. Assessment of citrate concentrations in citrus fruit-based juices and beverages: implications for management of hypocitraturic nephrolithiasis. J Endourol 2008;22(6):1359–66.

43. Wabner CL, Pak CY. Effect of orange juice consumption on urinary stone risk factors. J Urol 1993;149(6):1405–8.

44. Seltzer MA, Low RK, McDonald M, et al. Dietary manipulation with lemonade to treat hypocitraturic calcium nephrolithiasis. J Urol 1996;156(3):907–9.

45. Giannini S, Nobile M, Sartori L, et al. Acute effects of moderate dietary protein restriction in patients with idiopathic hypercalciuria and calcium nephrolithiasis. Am J Clin Nutr 1999;69(2):267–71.

46. Taylor EN, Fung TT, Curhan GC. DASH-style diet associates with reduced risk for kidney stones. J Am Soc Nephrol 2009;20(10):2253–9.

47. Taylor EN, Stampfer MJ, Mount DB, et al. DASH-style diet and 24-hour urine composition. Clin J Am Soc Nephrol 2010;5(12):2315–22.

48. Sakhaee K, Harvey JA, Padalino PK, et al. The potential role of salt abuse on the risk for kidney stone formation. J Urol 1993;150(2 Pt 1):310–2.

49. Domrongkitchaiporn S, Sopassathit W, Stitchantrakul W, et al. Schedule of taking calcium supplement and the risk of nephrolithiasis. Kidney Int 2004;65(5):1835–41.

50. Holmes RP, Assimos DG. The impact of dietary oxalate on kidney stone formation. Urol Res 2004;32(5):311–6.

51. Fink HA, Wilt TJ, Eidman KE, et al. Medical management to prevent recurrent nephrolithiasis in adults: a systematic review for an American college of physicians clinical guideline. Ann Intern Med 2013;158(7):535–43.

52. Borghi L, Meschi T, Guerra A, et al. Randomized prospective study of a nonthiazide diuretic, indapamide, in preventing calcium stone recurrences. J Cardiovasc Pharmacol 1993;22(Suppl 6):S78–86.

53. Ettinger B, Citron JT, Livermore B, et al. Chlorthalidone reduces calcium oxalate calculous recurrence but magnesium hydroxide does not. J Urol 1988;139(4):679–84.

54. Pak CY, Fuller C, Sakhaee K, et al. Long-term treatment of calcium nephrolithiasis with potassium citrate. J Urol 1985;134(1):11–9.

55. Coe FL. Hyperuricosuric calcium oxalate nephrolithiasis. Kidney Int 1978;13(5):418–26.

56. Barcelo P, Wuhl O, Servitge E, et al. Randomized double-blind study of potassium citrate in idiopathic hypocitraturic calcium nephrolithiasis. J Urol 1993;150(6):1761–4.

57. Hübner W, Porpaczy P. Treatment of caliceal calculi. Br J Urol 1990;66(1):9–11.

58. Leavitt DA, de la Rosette JJMCH, Hoenig DM. Strategies for nonmedical management of upper urinary tract calculi. In: Wein A, editor. Campbell-walsh urology. 11th edition. Philadelphia: Elsevier; 2016. p. 1235–59.e10. Available at: https://www.clinicalkey.com/#!/content/book/3-s2.0-B9781455775675000534. Accessed April 29, 2017.

59. Blandy JP, Singh M. The case for a more aggressive approach to staghorn stones. J Urol 1976;115(5):505–6.

60. Koga S, Arakaki Y, Matsuoka M, et al. Staghorn calculi–long-term results of management. Br J Urol 1991;68(2):122–4.

61. Segura JW, Preminger GM, Assimos DG, et al. Nephrolithiasis clinical guidelines panel summary report on the management of staghorn calculi. The American urological association nephrolithiasis clinical guidelines panel. J Urol 1994;151(6):1648–51.

62. Teichman JM, Long RD, Hulbert JC. Long-term renal fate and prognosis after staghorn calculus management. J Urol 1995;153(5):1403–7.
63. Mariappan P, Smith G, Moussa SA, et al. One week of ciprofloxacin before percutaneous nephrolithotomy significantly reduces upper tract infection and urosepsis: a prospective controlled study. BJU Int 2006;98(5):1075–9.
64. Bag S, Kumar S, Taneja N, et al. One week of nitrofurantoin before percutaneous nephrolithotomy significantly reduces upper tract infection and urosepsis: a prospective controlled study. Urology 2011;77(1):45–9.
65. de la Rosette J, Denstedt J, Geavlete P, et al. The clinical research office of the endourological society ureteroscopy global study: indications, complications, and outcomes in 11,885 patients. J Endourol 2014;28(2):131–9.
66. Sener NC, Imamoglu MA, Bas O, et al. Prospective randomized trial comparing shock wave lithotripsy and flexible ureterorenoscopy for lower pole stones smaller than 1 cm. Urolithiasis 2014;42(2):127–31.
67. Saw KC, Lingeman JE. Lesson 20: Management of calyceal stones. AUA Update Ser 1999;20:154–9.
68. Grasso M. Ureteropyeloscopic treatment of ureteral and intrarenal calculi. Urol Clin North Am 2000;27(4):623–31.
69. Resorlu B, Unsal A, Ziypak T, et al. Comparison of retrograde intrarenal surgery, shockwave lithotripsy, and percutaneous nephrolithotomy for treatment of medium-sized radiolucent renal stones. World J Urol 2013;31(6):1581–6.
70. Albala DM, Assimos DG, Clayman RV, et al. Lower pole I: a prospective randomized trial of extracorporeal shock wave lithotripsy and percutaneous nephrostolithotomy for lower pole nephrolithiasis-initial results. J Urol 2001;166(6):2072–80.
71. Murray MJ, Chandhoke PS, Berman CJ, et al. Outcome of extracorporeal shock-wave lithotripsy monotherapy for large renal calculi: effect of stone and collecting system surface areas and cost-effectiveness of treatment. J Endourol 1995;9(1):9–13.
72. Bryniarski P, Paradysz A, Zyczkowski M, et al. A randomized controlled study to analyze the safety and efficacy of percutaneous nephrolithotripsy and retrograde intrarenal surgery in the management of renal stones more than 2 cm in diameter. J Endourol 2012;26(1):52–7.
73. El-Assmy A, El-Nahas AR, Madbouly K, et al. Extracorporeal shock-wave lithotripsy monotherapy of partial staghorn calculi. Prognostic factors and long-term results. Scand J Urol Nephrol 2006;40(4):320–5.
74. Preminger GM, Tiselius H-G, Assimos DG, et al. 2007 guideline for the management of ureteral calculi. J Urol 2007;178(6):2418–34.
75. Morse RM, Resnick MI. Ureteral calculi: natural history and treatment in an era of advanced technology. J Urol 1991;145(2):263–5.
76. Yilmaz E, Batislam E, Basar MM, et al. The comparison and efficacy of 3 different alpha1-adrenergic blockers for distal ureteral stones. J Urol 2005;173(6):2010–2.
77. Singal RK, Denstedt JD. Contemporary management of ureteral stones. Urol Clin North Am 1997;24(1):59–70.
78. Maheshwari PN, Oswal AT, Andankar M, et al. Is antegrade ureteroscopy better than retrograde ureteroscopy for impacted large upper ureteral calculi? J Endourol 1999;13(6):441–4.
79. Stothers L, Lee LM. Renal colic in pregnancy. J Urol 1992;148(5):1383–7.
80. Butler EL, Cox SM, Eberts EG, et al. Symptomatic nephrolithiasis complicating pregnancy. Obstet Gynecol 2000;96(5 Pt 1):753–6.
81. Curhan GC. Epidemiology of stone disease. Urol Clin North Am 2007;34(3):287–93.

82. Lewis DF, Robichaux AG, Jaekle RK, et al. Urolithiasis in pregnancy. Diagnosis, management and pregnancy outcome. J Reprod Med 2003;48(1):28–32.
83. McAleer SJ, Loughlin KR. Nephrolithiasis and pregnancy. Curr Opin Urol 2004; 14(2):123–7.
84. Ross AE, Handa S, Lingeman JE, et al. Kidney stones during pregnancy: an investigation into stone composition. Urol Res 2008;36(2):99–102.
85. Deyoe LA, Cronan JJ, Breslaw BH, et al. New techniques of ultrasound and color Doppler in the prospective evaluation of acute renal obstruction. Do they replace the intravenous urogram? Abdom Imaging 1995;20(1):58–63.
86. Boridy IC, Maklad N, Sandler CM. Suspected urolithiasis in pregnant women: imaging algorithm and literature review. AJR Am J Roentgenol 1996;167(4):869–75.
87. Shokeir AA, Mahran MR, Abdulmaaboud M. Renal colic in pregnant women: role of renal resistive index. Urology 2000;55(3):344–7.
88. Elgamasy A, Elsherif A. Use of Doppler ultrasonography and rigid ureteroscopy for managing symptomatic ureteric stones during pregnancy. BJU Int 2010; 106(2):262–6.
89. Fulgham PF, Assimos DG, Pearle MS, et al. Clinical effectiveness protocols for imaging in the management of ureteral calculous disease: AUA technology assessment. J Urol 2013;189(4):1203–13.
90. White WM, Zite NB, Gash J, et al. Low-dose computed tomography for the evaluation of flank pain in the pregnant population. J Endourol 2007;21(11):1255–60.
91. American College of Obstetricians and Gynecologists' Committee on Obstetric Practice. Guidelines for diagnostic imaging during pregnancy and lactation. Obstet Gynecol 2016;127(2):e75–80.
92. Rodriguez PN, Klein AS. Management of urolithiasis during pregnancy. Surg Gynecol Obstet 1988;166(2):103–6.
93. Bailey G, Vaughan L, Rose C, et al. Perinatal outcomes with tamsulosin therapy for symptomatic urolithiasis. J Urol 2016;195(1):99–103.
94. Scarpa RM, De Lisa A, Usai E. Diagnosis and treatment of ureteral calculi during pregnancy with rigid ureteroscopes. J Urol 1996;155(3):875–7.
95. Frankenschmidt A, Sommerkamp H. Shock wave lithotripsy during pregnancy: a successful clinical experiment. J Urol 1998;159(2):501–2.

Frequent Urinary Tract Infection

Heidi Camus Turpen, MS, RD, MPAS, PA-C

KEYWORDS

- UTI • Recurrent UTI • Cystitis • Pyelonephritis • Bacteriuria

KEY POINTS

- No treatment is required for asymptomatic bacteriuria in nonpregnant individuals.
- Identifying uncomplicated versus complicated urinary tract infections (UTIs) will help to determine necessary further workup and treatment duration.
- Recurrent UTI workup should include physical examination, imaging, and cystoscopy.
- It is important to choose antibiotic choices and duration of treatment wisely.

Urinary tract infections (UTIs) are among the most common bacterial infections, hence one of the most common complaints encountered by primary care providers. By 26 years old, 1 in 3 women will have had at least one provider-diagnosed UTI, with an annual cost of $1.6 billion.[1] Approximately 50% to 80% of women will experience a UTI at some point in their lifetime, with 20% to 50% of women experiencing a recurrence.[2,3]

UTIs cause significant morbidity, affecting both men and women of all ages; however, women are significantly more likely to experience a UTI than men, mainly attributable to the anatomy of the female urethra, which is significantly shorter than the male urethra, thus an easier point of entry for bacterial pathogens. Most uropathogens originate in the rectal flora and colonize the perineum and periurethral tissues. Alterations in vaginal flora, specifically the loss of hydrogen peroxide–producing lactobacilli, as is seen in the postmenopausal state, may predispose women to colonization of the vaginal introitus with uropathogens, most commonly *Escherichia coli*.[4] This can predispose the postmenopausal female population to recurrent UTI. Other populations at increased risk of UTI include the elderly, pregnant women, patients with spinal cord injuries, indwelling or intermittent catheter users, patients with diabetes or multiple sclerosis, patients with acquired immunodeficiency disease syndrome or human immunodeficiency virus, and patients with underlying urologic abnormalities preventing adequate urinary drainage.[5] Incomplete urinary drainage provides a reservoir for bacterial colonization and growth. However, just because someone does not empty completely does not necessarily mean they will have an issue with UTI or bacteriuria.

The author has nothing to disclose.
Urology Department, University of Texas Southwestern Medical Center, 5323 Harry Hines Boulevard, Dallas, TX 75390, USA
E-mail address: Heidi.turpen@utsouthwestern.edu

Physician Assist Clin 3 (2018) 55–67
http://dx.doi.org/10.1016/j.cpha.2017.08.007
2405-7991/18/Published by Elsevier Inc.

Besides these populations, other risk factors for UTI include prior UTI; condom, diaphragm, or spermicide use; vaginal infection, trauma or manipulation; urinary tract instrumentation; sexual activity; obesity; and genetic susceptibility; that is, a mother with history of UTIs[6] (**Box 1**). There is also some evidence that recurrent UTIs could stem from intracellular populations of bacteria in the bladder urothelium that are quiescent for some time and may seed recurrent infection.[7]

Definitions

UTI: inflammatory response of the urothelium to bacterial that is associated with bacteriuria

Bacteriuria: presence of bacteria in the urine, which is normally sterile

Cystitis: inflammation of the bladder often caused by infection and usually accompanied by a clinical syndrome, which may include dysuria, frequency, urgency, and/or suprapubic pressure or pain

Pyelonephritis: inflammation of the kidney caused by infection and accompanied by a clinical syndrome, which may include fevers, chills, and flank pain

Catheter-associated UTI: culture proven UTI in a patient with an indwelling catheter, suprapubic tube, or on intermittent catheterization

Asymptomatic bacteriuria: bacteria detected in the urine without any associated symptoms in the patient

Sterile pyuria: the presence of WBC in the urine without bacteriuria

Recurrent UTI: greater than or equal to 2 infections within 6 months, or greater than or equal to 3 infections in 1 year

---

The clinical presentation of UTI can vary but may include dysuria, frequency, urgency, incontinence, hematuria, fever, suprapubic pain, nausea, vomiting, and malaise (**Box 2**). Additionally, when a patient has a suspected UTI with associated fever and flank pain, there is a higher suspicion that pyelonephritis may be present.

Pyelonephritis is less common than cystitis and has been estimated to occur more often in women at 3 to 4 cases per 10,000, as opposed to 1 to 2 cases per 10,000 in men in the outpatient population. Pyelonephritis occurs when bacteria ascends to

---

Box 1
Risk factors

- Female gender
- Sexually active
- Prior UTI
- Spermicide, condom, or diaphragm use
- Diabetes
- Obesity
- Trauma or manipulation
- Vaginal infection
- Family history (maternal history of UTI)
- First UTI at young age

Adapted from Foxman B. Urinary tract infection syndromes: occurrence, recurrence, bacteriology, risk factors, and disease burden. Infect Dis Clin North Am 2014;28(1):1–13.

> **Box 2**
> **Signs and symptoms**
>
> - Dysuria
> - Suprapubic pain or pressure
> - Flank pain
> - Fevers
> - Malaise
> - Nausea or vomiting
> - Urinary frequency and/or urgency
> - Hematuria

the kidneys from the bladder; however, it can also be caused by seeding of the kidneys from bacteremia or lymphatic infection. When a patient presents with fever, flank pain, costovertebral angle tenderness, and positive urine culture, pyelonephritis is likely present. Cystitis may or may not present with fevers or flank pain. Escherichia coli causes 80% of the cases in women and 70% of the cases in men.[8] Treatment of pyelonephritis usually ranges from 7 to 14 days, depending on if there are any urogenital abnormalities.[9] Pyelonephritis should be taken seriously because if this is left untreated or improperly treated, it may lead to sepsis. In approximately one-fourth of patients with sepsis, the focus of infection can be localized to the urinary tract.[10] Sepsis with the etiology found to be related to the genitourinary (GU) system is termed urosepsis.

It is important, in most cases, to objectively assess for infection of the urinary tract with urinalysis and urine culture rather than treating based on symptoms alone. Empirically treating patients based on their symptoms rather than urine cultures with reported sensitivities can lead to the development of multidrug-resistant bacteria and possibly incorrectly diagnosed recurrent UTIs. With a clean catch, midstream urine specimen, the Centers for Disease Control defines a UTI as 10^5 colony-forming units (CFU)/mL of bacteria grown in culture. With a catheterized specimen, the bacterial growth can be as low at 10^3 CFU/mL to qualify as a UTI. Gram-negative bacteria are isolated 75% to 95% of the time in uncomplicated UTIs,[11] with the most common uropathogen in premenopausal women being *Escherichia coli*, causing 80% to 85% of UTIs.[11,12] The most frequently isolated gram-positive uropathogens include *Staphylococcus saprophyticus*, *Enterococcus faecalis*, and *Streptococcus agalactiae* (GBS) (**Fig. 1**).[11] Women may be colonized with GBS in the vagina and/or rectum, therefore if there is any question as to if the GBS is actually causing cystitis, obtaining a catheterized specimen should clarify this.

There are scenarios when a clean catch, midstream urine collection is not possible to get a urine sample; for instance, in a patient with an indwelling urethral catheter, one who performs intermittent catheterizations, or one who has an ileal conduit. A urine sample should never be taken from a catheter or appliance bag. A new catheter should be placed and the urine acquired after this should be sent for evaluation. A clean catheterized specimen should be taken from patients who perform intermittent catheterization. Finally, in patients with urinary diversion, the stoma should be catheterized and this urine sample sent for culture.

UTIs can be described based on the anatomy of the urinary tract and/or the functional status of the patient. An uncomplicated UTI is one in which the patient's urinary tract is normal anatomically and functionally (**Box 3**).

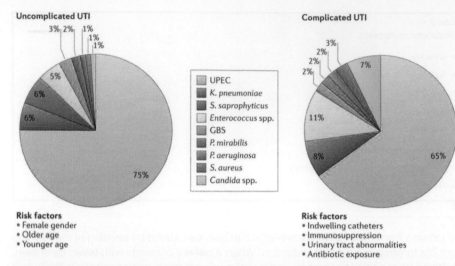

Fig. 1. Most common uropathogens in uncomplicated and complicated UTIs. (*From* Flores-Mireles AL, Walker JN, Caparon M, et al. Urinary tract infections: epidemiology, mechanisms of infection and treatment options. Nat Rev Microbiol 2015;13(5):270; with permission.)

Complicated UTIs occur in individuals with functional or structural abnormalities of the urinary tract. **Table 1** lists many causes leading to complicated UTIs, which may be obstructive, metabolic, functional, related to instrumentation, or other factors of the host[13,14]. Obstructive abnormalities, as well as functional abnormalities, such as a neurogenic bladder or vesicoureteral reflux, lead to the incomplete emptying of urine from the GU system, predisposing the individual to infection. The goal in these cases, while treating the infection, is to allow for adequate drainage of urine. Any foreign body in the GU system can allow for bacterial entrance to the bladder, as in catheterization, or provide a nidus of infection where bacteria tend to stick. If instrumentation, as in catheterization, is necessary, it is important to have specific timing set in place for exchange of these foreign bodies to attempt to reduce the risk of associated infection. For example, generally, indwelling urethral catheters should be exchanged every 4 weeks. The most common ureteral stents should be replaced every 3 to 6 months.

Catheter-associated UTI (CAUTI) is the most common nosocomial infection. Between 15% and 25% of patients in general hospitals may have a catheter in place

Box 3
Uncomplicated urinary tract infection
Immunocompetent
Minimal comorbidities
No known urologic abnormalities
Nonpregnant
Premenopausal
Data from Colgan R, Williams M. Diagnosis and treatment of acute uncomplicated cystitis. Am Fam Physician 2011;84(7):771–6.

Table 1
Structural and functional abnormalities of the genitourinary tract associated with complicated urinary tract infection

Obstructive	Prostatic hypertrophy
	Ureteric or urethral stricture
	Tumors
	Pelvicalyceal obstruction
	Urolithiasis
	Congenital abnormalities
	Renal cysts
Metabolic	Urolithiasis
	Diabetes
	Medullary sponge kidney
	Immunosuppression
	Renal failure
Functional	Neurogenic bladder (stroke, spinal cord injury, Parkinson disease, multiple sclerosis)
	Vesicoureteral reflux
Instrumentation	Indwelling urethral or suprapubic catheter
	Intermittent catheterization
	Ureteric stent
	Nephrostomy tube
	Cystoscopy
	Urodynamic bladder function study
Other	Ileal conduit
	Urologic surgery
Immunocompromised Host	
Pregnant	
Postmenopausal	
Men	

Data from Colgan R, Williams M. Diagnosis and treatment of acute uncomplicated cystitis. Am Fam Physician 2011;84(7):771–6; and Nicolle LE. A practical guide to antimicrobial management of complicated urinary tract infection. Drugs Aging 2001;18(4):243–54.

at one point during their stay.[15] Up to 50% of patients requiring an indwelling catheter for 5 days or longer will develop bacteriuria or candiduria.[16] The incidence of this being reported at approximately 10% per day.[16] Initiatives to reduce the CAUTI are not only important for patient health but also important from a financial standpoint because hospital-acquired CAUTIs are not reimbursed by Medicare. Reminder systems are one method to prompt removal of unnecessary catheters and this has been found to reduce the rate of CAUTI by 52%.[17] Sterile and clean intermittent catheterization have an incidence of bacteriuria ranging from 1% to 3% per catheterization.[18] Thus, if possible, clean intermittent catheterization is the preferred method for incomplete bladder emptying. Urinary incontinence is not a valid reason to have a catheter in place.

When it comes to noting bacteriuria, whether a patient has an indwelling catheter or not, it is important to define whether a patient is symptomatic or asymptomatic, with the former requiring treatment but not the latter. The prevalence of asymptomatic bacteriuria varies based on gender, age, and comorbidities, with the highest prevalence in patients with indwelling catheters, and in women more than men. Asymptomatic bacteriuria should generally not be treated with antimicrobials. There are certain exceptions to this, including screening pregnant women, during evaluation before urologic procedures, and possibly during the first few years after transplant surgery in a case by case basis. However, some evidence shows there is no benefit to treating asymptomatic bacteriuria in the short-term or long-term for transplanted patients.[19] Pregnant women with bacteriuria are more likely to have premature delivery and to deliver infants with low birth weight; treatment in this population has decreased the frequency of this adverse outcome.[20,21] Additionally, during early pregnancy, women with asymptomatic bacteriuria have a 20-fold to 30-fold increased risk of developing pyelonephritis during pregnancy.[22–29] The proposed mechanisms causing this include progesterone-induced smooth muscle relaxation of ureteral peristalsis and, later in pregnancy, the mechanical compression of the ureter, which causes incomplete drainage of urine. Treatment of UTI or asymptomatic bacteriuria in the pregnant woman should be done in close conjunction with the individual's obstetrician.

RECURRENT URINARY TRACT INFECTION

Recurrent UTIs may be either due to reinfection or relapse. Reinfection is a new UTI with a different pathogen than the pretherapy isolate. A relapse is another infection with the same pathogen as in pretherapy. Complicating matters, reinfection may occur with the same organism and, in this case, make it impossible to distinguish between them. If infection with the same organism persists, it is important to decipher if a previous infection was completely and appropriately treated. If it was, and seems to symptomatically persist, referral to a urology provider is warranted. If more than 2 weeks have passed since treatment and the same organism is present, this is considered to be reinfection.

Recurrent UTIs refers to greater than or equal to 2 infections within 6 months, or greater than or equal to 3 infections in 1 year. Most recurrence is thought to represent reinfection. Relapse, however, is important to identify because it may be due to a nidus of infection in the urinary tract or other structural abnormality, which may warrant surgical intervention.

WORKUP OF RECURRENT URINARY TRACT INFECTION

For patients with recurrent UTI, it is important to initiate workup to evaluate for any reversible risk factors that could be leading to the recurrent infection. Specifically, the urinary tract must be evaluated for anatomic or structural abnormalities. The evaluation may include:

- Physical examination
  - Female GU exam to check for presence of atrophic vaginitis and/or prolapse
  - Postvoid residual bladder scan to evaluate for bladder emptying
- Imaging
  - Renal ultrasound (US) to identify large calculi, hydronephrosis, perirenal abscess, and postvoid residual
  - Computed tomography or MRI, which are more sensitive than US, to identify renal and perirenal abscesses, radiolucent calculi, and acute focal bacterial nephritis
  - Voiding cystourethrogram to evaluate for vesicoureteral reflux and urethral diverticulum
- Cystoscopy
  - Performed at an urologic office, to evaluate bladder for foreign objects, calculi, tumors, trigonitis, and obvious pockets of infection in the urothelium.

PREVENTION STRATEGIES AND TREATMENT

Most uncomplicated UTIs can be treated with antimicrobials for 3 to 5 days depending on the agent used. The American Urological Association recommends first-line therapy to be nitrofurantoin or trimethoprim-sulfamethoxazole (TMP-SMX). In a 2015 update from the American Urogynecologic Society, it is recommended that for women with uncomplicated UTIs, fluoroquinolone antibiotics should not be first-line treatment due to their higher risk of adverse events, including bacterial resistance. Fluoroquinolones should be saved for treatment of UTIs in individuals who cannot receive nitrofurantoin, TMP-SMX, or fosfomycin (Table 2). Urine cultures obtained should provide antimicrobial susceptibility profiles for the uropathogen so that the appropriate antibiotic is chosen.

Several strategies have been routinely used to attempt to decrease recurrent UTIs. Recommended behavioral changes include avoiding spermicides and diaphragm use, which can alter the vaginal flora. Postcoital voiding is reasonable although not much data exist to routinely support this to reduce risk of UTI, however, there is no harm in doing so. Antimicrobial prophylaxis has been shown to be highly effective in reducing recurrent UTI during the prophylaxis treatment period in women with anatomically and functionally normal urinary tracts.[30,31] This is done on a daily basis versus postcoitally, depending on the patient profile. Many women are able to associate their infections with intercourse and there is evidence that in premenopausal women there is no difference in the rate of UTIs if prophylaxis is taken postcotally versus daily.[32] In patients who cannot pinpoint an infection relationship with intercourse, antibiotic prophylaxis regimens of 6 to 12 months' duration versus placebo have shown a significantly reduced risk of clinical recurrence of 85%. However, after antibiotic prophylaxis has ceased, there is no significantly reduced infection rate in the prophylaxis-treated individuals.[33] Regardless, for many individuals, this infection-free time is life-changing.

Options for continuous or pericoital antibiotic prophylaxis should be chosen based on an individual's UTI history and susceptibility patterns of their infections. Options include

- TMP-SMX 40 mg/200 mg daily
- TMP-SMX 80 mg/400 mg daily
- Trimethoprim 100 mg daily
- Nitrofurantoin 50 mg daily
- Nitrofurantoin 100 mg daily
- Cefaclor 250 mg daily
- Cephalexin 125 mg daily
- Cephalexin 250 mg daily

Table 2	
Infectious Disease Society of America drugs commonly used for cystitis in women	
First-line therapy	Nitrofurantoin 100 mg bid × 5 d
	TMP-SMX 1 DS tablet (160 mg/800 mg) bid × 3 d
Second-line therapy	Ciprofloxacin 250 mg q 12 h × 3 d or 500 mg q day × 3 d
Other commonly used antibiotics for inpatient use	Ceftriaxone 1 g q 24 h
	Zosyn 3.375 g q 6 h or higher for *Pseudomonas aeruginosa* dosing
	Tobramycin 3 mg/kg/d

- Norfloxacin 200 mg daily
- Ciprofloxacin 125 mg daily.

In reliable patients with a well-documented history of cultures, self-start therapy may be considered cautiously. There is evidence that this method can be accurate in self-diagnosis greater than 85% to 95% of the time, with effective treatment of the UTI.[34–36] If symptoms persist or worsen, however, these patients should have a low threshold to contact their provider for appropriate evaluation, including urine culture. Bacterial resistance may have emerged, or there may be some other cause for their symptoms.

In postmenopausal women, topical vaginal estrogen helps to normalize the vaginal flora and reduce the risk of UTI. This same effect is not always found when taking oral estrogen.[37] When using vaginal estrogen, the vaginal pH and flora becomes more favorable. Vaginal pH is lower, more lactobacilli are present in vaginal cultures, and less vaginal Enterobacteriaceae is present.[38] This leads to decreased numbers of uropathogens traveling from vagina to urethra to bladder.

There is mixed evidence regarding cranberry supplementation and its effect on UTI. Laboratory studies have shown that cranberry may inhibit adherence of pathogens to the uroepithelial cells.[39,40] However a 2012 Cochrane review evaluating cranberry products suggests that it is no more effective than placebo.[41] In most cases, it likely is not harmful to add a cranberry supplement in an attempt to ward off UTI; however, there are some medication interactions with cranberry, including with warfarin, which should be considered when taking this supplement.

Probiotics containing *Lactobacillus* are safe and may be effective in preventing recurrent UTIs in adult women; however, more randomized controlled trials are required before a definitive recommendation can be made.[42] The theory behind this is similar to the vaginal estrogen treatment in postmenopausal women. The presence of lactobacilli in the vaginal flora is more likely to decrease the presence of uropathogens.

ANTIBIOTIC STEWARDSHIP

When it comes to treating UTIs, specifically recurrent UTIs, it is important to be diligent in antibiotic use to prevent resistance patterns of uropathogens. Antimicrobials that affect the gastrointestinal flora more significantly (trimethoprim, TMP-SMX, quinolones, and ampicillin), have shown increased rates of antimicrobial resistance.[43,44] There is also a geographic variation in resistance patterns. Resistance to TMP-SMX, a currently recommended first-line therapy for outpatient cystitis in women, is around 18% to 22%, depending on region.[45] **Table 3** shows multiple antimicrobial agents and the uropathogen that they treat.

- A few points to note regarding many antimicrobial agents used in the treatment of UTIs:
- Nitrofurantoin is rapidly excreted from the urine but does not obtain therapeutic levels in most body tissues; therefore, it is not to be used for pyelonephritis. Acquired bacterial resistance is very low.
- TMP-SMX has increased resistance patterns. It can be used for treatment of pyelonephritis if the uropathogen is known to be susceptible.

Fosfomycin is an oral bactericidal agent with activity against most urinary tract pathogens, particularly *Escherichia coli*, *Citrobacter*, *Enterobacter*, *Klebsiella*, *Serratia*, and *Enterococcus* spp. It is primarily excreted unchanged in the urine. Following a single 3 g oral dose, urinary concentration remains high for 24 to 48 hours, which is sufficient

Table 3
Reliable coverage of antimicrobials used in the treatment of urinary tract infections of commonly encountered pathogens

Antimicrobial Agent or Class	Gram-Positive Pathogens	Gram-Negative Pathogens
Amoxicillin or ampicillin (po)	Streptococcus Enterococci	Proteus mirabilis
Amoxicillin with clavulanate (po)	Streptococcus Enterococci	P mirabilis Klebsiella spp
Ampicillin with sulbactam (IV)	Staphylococcus (not MRSA) Enterococci	P mirabilis Haemophilus influenzae, Klebsiella spp
Antistaphylococcal penicillins	Streptococcus Staphylococcus (not MRSA)	None
Antipseudomonal penicillins	Streptococcus Enterococci	Most, including Pseudomonas aeruginosa
First-generation cephalosporins (po)	Streptococcus Staphylococcus (not MRSA)	Escherichia coli P mirabilis Klebsiella spp
Second-generation cephalosporins (cefuroxime, IV; cefaclor, po)	Streptococcus Staphylococcus (not MRSA)	Escherichia coli, P mirabilis H influenzae, Klebsiella spp
Second-generation cephalosporins (cefoxitin, cefotetan, IV)	Streptococcus	Escherichia coli, Proteus spp (including indole-positive) H influenzae, Klebsiella spp
Third-generation cephalosporins (ceftriaxone, IV; cefpodoxime, po)	Streptococcus Staphylococcus (not MRSA)	Most, excluding P aeruginosa
Third-generation cephalosporins (ceftazidime, IV)	Streptococcus	Most, including P aeruginosa
Aztreonam (IV)	None	Most, including P aeruginosa
Aminoglycosides (IV)	Staphylococcus (urine)	Most, including P aeruginosa
Fluoroquinolones (po, IV)	Streptococcus	Most, including P aeruginosa
Nitrofurantoin (po)	Staphylococcus (not MRSA) Enterococci	Many Enterobacteriaceae (not Providencia, Serratia, Acinetobacter) Klebsiella spp
Fosfomycin (po)	Enterococci	Most Enterobacteriaceae
TMP-SMX (po)	Streptococcus Staphylococcus	Most Enterobacteriaceae (not P aeruginosa)
Vancomycin (IV)	All, including MRSA	None

Abbreviations: IV, intravenous; PO, by mouth.
Adapted from Wein AJ, Kavoussi LR, Partin AW, et al. Campbell Walsh Urology. 11th edition. Philadelphia: Elsevier; 2016; with permission.

to inhibit most uropathogens.[46] It is effective against extended-spectrum beta-lactamase (ESBL) producer, vancomycin-resistant enterococci (VRE), and methicillin-resistant *Staphylococcus aureu*s (MRSA).[47,48] Fosfomycin is not reported on sensitivity reports but is important to keep in mind when resistant uropathogens are encountered because it can be the last oral option before parenteral therapy is needed. However, cost can be a barrier.

Fluoroquinolones has increasing resistance among gram-negative uropathogens and are no longer recommended as first-line for uncomplicated cystitis.[49] Use of fluoroquinolones has been linked to subsequent infection with MRSA and fluoroquinolone-resistant gram-negative bacilli.[50]

Cephalosporins show activity against Enterobacteriaceae; however, not against ESBL-producing uropathogens.[51] It is an appropriate choice for treatment of pyelonephritis in patients not requiring hospitalization; however, it is important to know the prevalence of resistance to fluoroquinolones in the community. It is recommended not to use this if the resistance is thought to exceed 10%.[52] Use of broad-spectrum cephalosporins has been linked to subsequent infection with VRE, ESBL *Klebsiella*, beta-lactam–resistant *Acinetobacter* spp, and *Clostridium difficile*.[50]

Aminopenicillins, including amoxicillin and ampicillin, have a high prevalence of antimicrobial resistance.[52] Effects on vaginal flora include vaginal candidiasis. Augmentin, which is the addition of the beta-lactamase inhibitor, clavulanate, to amoxicillin, improves activity against beta-lactamase–producing bacteria.

Aminoglycosides have a low prevalence of resistance. Resistance emergence during therapy is rare.[53,54] There are fewer adverse effects overall with aminoglycoside treatment versus beta-lactams; however, nephrotoxicity is significantly more common.[55]

STERILE PYURIA

Urine dipstick testing evaluates urine specific gravity, pH, leukocyte esterase, nitrites, bilirubin, protein, glucose, and blood. Pyuria is defined as the presence of greater than or equal to 10 white blood cells (WBC)/mm^3 in a urine sample or greater than or equal to 3 WBC/high power field (HPF) of unspun urine.[56] Sterile pyuria is the presence of WBC in the urine without bacteriuria. In symptomatic women with pyuria but without significant bacteriuria, there could be a low bacterial count, less than 10^5 CFU/mL, or infection with atypical organisms such as *Chlamydia trachomatis*.[57] Other causes of sterile pyuria include contamination of the sample by vaginal leukocytes from vaginal secretions, contamination from sterilizing solution used to clean meatus, chronic interstitial nephritis, nephrolithiasis, uroepithelial tumor, intra-abdominal inflammatory process adjacent to bladder, and/or infection with atypical organisms (*Chlamydia trachomatis*, *Neisseria gonorrhoeae*, Herpes Simplex Virus 2 (HSV2), *Ureaplasma urealyticum*, and tuberculosis).[58] Most commonly, sterile pyuria seen in women could be contamination related to vaginal secretions. In this scenario, it is best to get a catheterized specimen to evaluate for leukocytes with microscopy before referring the patient to a urology provider (**Table 4**).

Table 4 Evaluation of sterile pyuria	
Comprehensive metabolic panel	Chlamydia, ureaplasma, mycoplasma testing
Complete blood count	Urine cytology or other urothelial tumor marker
Formal urinalysis	Computed tomography urogram
Urine culture for bacteria, fungus, and mycobacteria (3 consecutive early AM samples for acid-fast staining and mycobacterial culture and sensitivities)	Cystoscopy

Adapted from Foxman B. Urinary tract infection syndromes: occurrence, recurrence, bacteriology, risk factors, and disease burden. Infect Dis Clin North Am 2014;28(1):1–13; with permission

REFERENCES

1. Foxman B, Barlow R, D'Arcy H, et al. Urinary tract infection: self-reported incidence and associated costs. Ann Epidemiol 2000;10(8):509–15.
2. Ikäheimo R, Siitonen A, Heiskanen T, et al. Recurrence of urinary tract infection in a primary care setting: analysis of a 1-year follow-up of 179 women. Clin Infect Dis 1996;22(1):91–9.
3. Stamm WE, McKevitt M, Roberts PL, et al. Natural history of recurrent urinary tract infections in women. Rev Infect Dis 1991;13(1):77–84.
4. Gupta K, Stamm WE. Pathogenesis and management of recurrent urinary tract infections in women. World J Urol 1999;17(6):415–20.
5. Foxman B. Epidemiology of urinary tract infections: incidence, morbidity, and economic costs. Am J Med 2002;113(1):5–13.
6. Foxman B. Urinary tract infection syndromes: occurrence, recurrence, bacteriology, risk factors, and disease burden. Infect Dis Clin North Am 2014;28(1): 1–13.
7. Rosen DA, Hooton TM, Stamm WE, et al. Detection of intracellular bacterial communities in human urinary tract infection. PLoS Med 2007;4(12):e329.
8. Czaja CA, Scholes D, Hooton TM, et al. Population-based epidemiologic analysis of acute pyelonephritis. Clin Infect Dis 2007;45(3):273–80.
9. Eliakim-Raz N, Yahav D, Paul M, et al. Duration of antibiotic treatment for acute pyelonephritis and septic urinary tract infection– 7 days or less versus longer treatment: systematic review and meta-analysis of randomized controlled trials. J Antimicrob Chemother 2013;68(10):2183–91.
10. Kalra OP, Raizada A. Approach to a patient with urosepsis. J Glob Infect Dis 2009;1(1):57–63.
11. Kline KA, Lewis AL. Gram-positive uropathogens, polymicrobial urinary tract infection, and the emerging microbiota of the urinary tract. Microbiol Spectr 2016;4(2). http://dx.doi.org/10.1128/microbiolspec.UTI-0012-2012.
12. Fihn SD. Clinical practice. Acute uncomplicated urinary tract infection in women. N Engl J Med 2003;349(3):259–66.
13. Colgan R, Williams M. Diagnosis and treatment of acute uncomplicated cystitis. Am Fam Physician 2011;84(7):771–6.
14. Nicolle LE. A practical guide to antimicrobial management of complicated urinary tract infection. Drugs Aging 2001;18(4):243–54.
15. Warren JW. Catheter-associated urinary tract infections. Int J Antimicrob Agents 2001;17(4):299–303.
16. Tambyah PA, Maki DG. Catheter-associated urinary tract infection is rarely symptomatic: a prospective study of 1497 catheterized patients. Arch Intern Med 2000;160(5):678–82.
17. Meddings J, Rogers MAM, Macy M, et al. Systematic review and meta-analysis: reminder systems to reduce catheter-associated urinary tract infections and urinary catheter use in hospitalized patients. Clin Infect Dis 2010;51(5):550–60.
18. Warren JW. Catheter-associated urinary tract infections. Infect Dis Clin North Am 1997;11(3):609–22.
19. Green H, Rahamimov R, Goldberg E, et al. Consequences of treated versus untreated asymptomatic bacteriuria in the first year following kidney transplantation: retrospective observational study. Eur J Clin Microbiol Infect Dis 2013;32(1): 127–31.

20. Mittendorf R, Williams MA, Kass EH. Prevention of preterm delivery and low birth weight associated with asymptomatic bacteriuria. Clin Infect Dis 1992;14(4):927–32.

21. Romero R, Oyarzun E, Mazor M, et al. Meta-analysis of the relationship between asymptomatic bacteriuria and preterm delivery/low birth weight. Obstet Gynecol 1989;73(4):576–82.

22. Elder HA, Santamarina BAG, Smith S, et al. The natural history of asymptomatic bacteriuria during pregnancy: the effect of tetracycline on the clinical course and the outcome of pregnancy. Am J Obstet Gynecol 1971;111(3):441–62.

23. Brumfitt W. The effects of bacteriuria in pregnancy on maternal and fetal health. Kidney Int Suppl 1975;4:S113–9.

24. Wren BG. Subclinical renal infection and prematurity. Med J Aust 1969;2(12):596–600.

25. Gilstrap LC, Leveno KJ, Cunningham FG, et al. Renal infection and pregnancy outcome. Am J Obstet Gynecol 1981;141(6):709–16.

26. Little PJ. The incidence of urinary infection in 5000 pregnant women. Lancet 1966;2(7470):925–8.

27. Leblanc AL, Mcganity WJ. The impact of bacteriuria in pregnancy; A survey of 1300 pregnant patients. Tex Rep Biol Med 1964;22:336–47.

28. Kincaid-Smith P, Bullen M. Bacteriuria in pregnancy. Lancet 1965;1(7382):395–9.

29. Savage WE, Hajj SN, Kass EH. Demographic and prognostic characteristics of bacteriuria in pregnancy. Medicine (Baltimore) 1967;46(5):385–407.

30. Stamm WE, Hooton TM. Management of Urinary Tract Infections in Adults. N Engl J Med 1993;329(18):1328–34.

31. Nicolle LE. Prophylaxis: recurrent urinary tract infection in women. Infection 1992;20(Suppl 3):S203–5 [discussion: S206–10].

32. Melekos MD, Asbach HW, Gerharz E, et al. Post-intercourse versus daily ciprofloxacin prophylaxis for recurrent urinary tract infections in premenopausal women. J Urol 1997;157(3):935–9.

33. Masson P, Matheson S, Webster AC, et al. Meta-analyses in prevention and treatment of urinary tract infections. Infect Dis Clin North Am 2009;23(2):355–85.

34. Gupta K, Hooton TM, Roberts PL, et al. Patient-initiated treatment of uncomplicated recurrent urinary tract infections in young women. Ann Intern Med 2001;135(1):9–16.

35. Wong ES, McKevitt M, Running K, et al. Management of recurrent urinary tract infections with patient-administered single-dose therapy. Ann Intern Med 1985;102(3):302–7.

36. Schaeffer AJ, Stuppy BA. Efficacy and safety of self-start therapy in women with recurrent urinary tract infections. J Urol 1999;161(1):207–11.

37. Beerepoot MAJ, Geerlings SE, van Haarst EP, et al. Nonantibiotic prophylaxis for recurrent urinary tract infections: a systematic review and meta-analysis of randomized controlled trials. J Urol 2013;190(6):1981–9.

38. Raz R, Stamm WE. A controlled trial of intravaginal estriol in postmenopausal women with recurrent urinary tract infections. N Engl J Med 1993;329(11):753–6.

39. Schmidt DR, Sobota AE. An examination of the anti-adherence activity of cranberry juice on urinary and nonurinary bacterial isolates. Microbios 1988;55(224–225):173–81.

40. Sobota AE. Inhibition of bacterial adherence by cranberry juice: potential use for the treatment of urinary tract infections. J Urol 1984;131(5):1013–6.

41. Jepson RG, Williams G, Craig JC. Cranberries for preventing urinary tract infections. Cochrane Database Syst Rev 2012;(10):CD001321. John Wiley & Sons, Ltd; 2012.
42. Grin PM, Kowalewska PM, Alhazzan W, et al. Lactobacillus for preventing recurrent urinary tract infections in women: meta-analysis. Can J Urol 2013;20(1):6607–14.
43. Mavromanolakis E, Maraki S, Samonis G, et al. Effect of norfloxacin, trimethoprim-sulfamethoxazole and nitrofurantoin on fecal flora of women with recurrent urinary tract infections. J Chemother 1997;9(3):203–7.
44. Sullivan Å, Edlund C, Nord CE. Effect of antimicrobial agents on the ecological balance of human microflora. Lancet Infect Dis 2001;1(2):101–14.
45. Gupta K, Sahm DF, Mayfield D, et al. Antimicrobial resistance among uropathogens that cause community-acquired urinary tract infections in women: a nationwide analysis. Clin Infect Dis 2001;33(1):89–94.
46. Patel SS, Balfour JA, Bryson HM. Fosfomycin tromethamine. Drugs 1997;53(4):637–56.
47. Falagas ME, Kastoris AC, Kapaskelis AM, et al. Fosfomycin for the treatment of multidrug-resistant, including extended-spectrum beta-lactamase producing, Enterobacteriaceae infections: a systematic review. Lancet Infect Dis 2010;10(1):43–50.
48. Popovic M, Steinort D, Pillai S, et al. Fosfomycin: an old, new friend? Eur J Clin Microbiol Infect Dis 2010;29(2):127–42.
49. Bouchillon S, Hoban DJ, Badal R, et al. Fluoroquinolone resistance among gram-negative urinary tract pathogens: global smart program results, 2009-2010. Open Microbiol J 2012;6:74–8.
50. Paterson DL. "Collateral damage" from cephalosporin or quinolone antibiotic therapy. Clin Infect Dis 2004;38(Supplement_4):S341–5.
51. Pitout JD, Laupland KB. Extended-spectrum β-lactamase-producing Enterobacteriaceae: an emerging public-health concern. Lancet Infect Dis 2008;8(3):159–66.
52. Gupta K, Hooton TM, Naber KG, et al. International clinical practice guidelines for the treatment of acute uncomplicated cystitis and pyelonephritis in women: a 2010 update by the Infectious Diseases Society of America and the European Society for Microbiology and Infectious Diseases. Clin Infect Dis 2011;52(5):e103–20.
53. Pfaller MA, Jones RN, Doern GV, et al. Bacterial pathogens isolated from patients with bloodstream infection: frequencies of occurrence and antimicrobial susceptibility patterns from the SENTRY antimicrobial surveillance program (United States and Canada, 1997). Antimicrob Agents Chemother 1998;42(7):1762–70.
54. Jones RN, Sader HS, Beach ML. Contemporary in vitro spectrum of activity summary for antimicrobial agents tested against 18569 strains non-fermentative Gram-negative bacilli isolated in the SENTRY Antimicrobial Surveillance Program (1997–2001). Int J Antimicrob Agents 2003;22(6):551–6.
55. Vidal L, Gafter-Gvili A, Borok S, et al. Efficacy and safety of aminoglycoside monotherapy: systematic review and meta-analysis of randomized controlled trials. J Antimicrob Chemother 2007;60(2):247–57.
56. Horan TC, Andrus M, Dudeck MA. CDC/NHSN surveillance definition of health care–associated infection and criteria for specific types of infections in the acute care setting. Am J Infect Control 2008;36(5):309–32.
57. Stamm WE. Measurement of pyuria and its relation to bacteriuria. Am J Med 1983;75(1B):53–8.
58. Wise GJ, Schlegel PN. Sterile Pyuria. N Engl J Med 2015;372(11):1048–54.

Female Urinary Incontinence

Gwendolyn Brooke Zilinskas, MMS, PA-C

KEYWORDS

- Female incontinence • Stress incontinence • Urgency incontinence
- Mixed incontinence

KEY POINTS

- This article is an overview of the etiology, history, and physical examination findings, diagnostic testing, and treatment of women with various types of incontinence.
- Urinary incontinence is a common, yet underdiagnosed medical condition that increases in prevalence with each decade of life.
- Urinary incontinence can be subdivided into stress incontinence, urgency incontinence, functional incontinence, and extra-urethral incontinence among others. There are also mixed incontinence which can include multiple subtypes.
- Urinary incontinence can often be diagnosed with a thorough patient history and physical exam, including a pelvic exam. However, when the diagnosis is still unclear or treatment is not working there are several diagnostic studies that are available to better understand the clinical situation.

Urinary incontinence in women is a significant problem in health care today. Estimates of its prevalence vary greatly from 26% to 61% of women including all age groups and is often underdiagnosed.[1–3] Patients are often reluctant to discuss their urinary incontinence because of embarrassment, feeling like this is a normal part of aging, lack of understanding treatment options, and other factors. It is also known that incontinence increases with age with the most affected population being those living with cognitive or functional impairments and those persons living in a nursing home.[4,5]

Despite this condition being significantly underreported, it is important to ask patients about their bladder habits and any incontinence, as it significantly impacts quality of life. Patients who suffer from incontinence have more depression, anxiety, and social isolation.[6] It affects sexual intimacy and overall sexual function. It is also associated with an increased caregiver burden and often is the final symptom resulting in admission to a nursing home.[7]

The authors have nothing to disclose.
Department of Urology, The University of Texas Southwestern Medical Center, 5323 Harry Hines Boulevard, Dallas, TX 75390, USA
E-mail address: brooke.zilinskas@utsouthwestern.edu

Physician Assist Clin 3 (2018) 69–82
http://dx.doi.org/10.1016/j.cpha.2017.08.010
2405-7991/18/© 2017 Elsevier Inc. All rights reserved.

TYPES OF URINARY INCONTINENCE

Incontinence is defined as the involuntary loss of urine. This could be preempted by various stimuli.

Stress Urinary Incontinence

Stress urinary incontinence (SUI) refers to the loss of urine preceded by an increase in the intra-abdominal pressure. The pressure in the abdomen becomes greater than the resistance of the external sphincter muscle and leakage occurs. These forces can include coughing, sneezing, laughing, changing positions, and lifting. Women can also be prone to stress incontinence with increased abdominal weight and pregnancy. Additionally, forces that decrease the strength of the external sphincter increase the risk of stress urinary incontinence; therefore, weakening of the pelvic floor musculature after pelvic trauma, pelvic surgery, lower back surgery, and postmenopausal status contribute to the development and worsening of SUI.

Urgency Urinary Incontinence

Urgency urinary incontinence (UUI) can include leakage and also the urgency to void without leakage or overactive bladder (OAB). OAB occurs when there is an abnormal contraction of the detrusor muscle and the brain is triggered that it is time to urinate. If the contraction of the bladder muscle is greater than the resistance of the external urinary sphincter, then leakage will occur. These contractions can occur in neurologically intact patients and also in patients in whom there has been some disturbance in the bladder-to-brain connection (ie, multiple sclerosis, spinal cord injury, Parkinson disease, cerebrovascular accident, and others).

Mixed Incontinence

As one can assume, it is common that patients are bothered by more than one form of incontinence, and the more bothersome form can often be difficult to tease out of the patient history. Many patients who have SUI at baseline learn that if they void more often, they are less likely to have incontinence and therefore report frequency and urgency in their history. Patients with urgency incontinence may not feel an urge until they go to stand up from a chair after several hours of sitting down, and once they feel that urge, they find themselves running to the restroom with incontinence along the way. Additionally, many patients have both mechanisms of incontinence, and it may require treatment of one type of incontinence first. After the first treatment has been optimized, additional treatment can be offered if the patient is still not pleased with her level of leakage. Although it is acceptable to try to give the patient with mixed incontinence a prescription for her urgency incontinence, this may not be effective if the patient leaks with a low leak point pressure. This means that the bladder will leak with very little urine present if a stress incontinence trigger occurs. In these situations, advanced bladder testing is important in guiding clinician treatment and patient expectations.

Functional Urinary Incontinence

Functional Urinary Incontinence may have some components of SUI and urgency urinary incontinence, but the dominant problem is that the patient is not mentally able to understand that they need to urinate or physically able to get to the restroom in time. These patients may have congenital or acquired cognitive defects or physical challenges that cause them to need assistive devices (eg, walkers, wheelchairs).

Continuous Urinary Incontinence

Continuous urinary incontinence is a complex form of urinary incontinence and must be thoroughly evaluated. As the name suggests, continuous urinary incontinence is high-volume leakage without any known preemptive event. It is most commonly seen in a woman with previous pelvic surgery or radiation who has persistent urinary incontinence in the form of a vesico-vaginal fistula in which there is a connection from the bladder into the vagina causing persistent incontinence. Despite the frustration women feel, it is important to wait 10 to 12 weeks after the pelvic surgery so that the tissues heal before surgically repairing the fistula. Treatment is surgical and can be done through a vaginal, open abdominal, or robotic approach.

Overflow Urinary Incontinence

As the name suggests, overflow urinary incontinence refers to an inability to empty the bladder and retaining such large amounts of urine that any more urine created will cause the bladder to overflow out the urethra. These patients may have some element of obstruction from prior surgery or tumor, severe pelvic organ prolapse, or stricture. However, they may also have developed an underactive or neurogenic bladder over time, and their detrusor simply cannot generate enough of a contraction to allow the patient to void. The treatment of these patients first involves preservation of the upper tracts by draining the bladder. Patients can be taught to clean intermittent catheterization, but if they are unwilling to learn or considered unreliable, then a Foley catheter needs to be placed. Upper tract imaging, such as a renal ultrasound scan, and creatinine level should be considered at the time of catheter placement to ensure the kidneys are functioning and there is no upper tract drainage problem in the form of hydronephrosis. The patient should be counseled about postobstructive diuresis and admitted to the hospital if they are not reliable in measuring their intake and output at home. Medications known to cause urinary retention should be stopped if possible, and urodynamic testing should be considered in patients who can participate in the testing **(Table 1)**.[8]

EVALUATION OF THE INCONTINENT PATIENT

Evaluation of a woman with urinary incontinence should start with a thorough patient history. It is important to define and quantify the leakage of urine both to understand the cause and to document that any treatment is improving the symptoms. In the incontinent patient, providers should ask the patient to describe her leakage. It should also be noted the daytime urinary frequency, how often the patient wakes at night to void, and if there is ever any sense of urgency related to urination. Furthermore, a description of the patient's voiding habits should be obtained. Specific voiding information includes if there is any hesitancy in initiating urination, if the urine stream seems strong or weak, if the flow is steady or intermittent, and if the patient feels that they fully empty their bladder. Additional questions include if the patient needs to strain at any time during voiding, if they find themselves leaning forward or getting into other positions to assist with urine flow, and if there is any pain with urination (excluding discomfort associated with urinary tract infections).

When specifically discussing incontinence, it is important to find out how long the problem has been occurring; if it is getting worse, better, or stable over time; and any aggravating factors that cause the leakage. Additionally, the patient needs to explain how much leakage occurs each time (ie, if it is a few drops of urine or if it is a large gush). Although it is sometimes difficult to quantify, providers can sometimes get a sense of the amount of leakage during an incontinence episode by asking the

Table 1
Medications associated with urinary retention

Sympathomimetics (α-adrenergic agents)	• Ephedrine (Marax, Tedral) • Phenylephrine HCl (Neo-Synephrine) • Phenylpropanolamine HCl (Conlac) • Pseudoephedrine HCl (Sudafed, Actifed)
Sympathomimetics (β-adrenergic agents)	• Isoproterenol • Metaproterenol • Terbutaline
Antidepressants	• Imipramine (Tofranil) • Nortriptyline (Aventyl) • Amitriptyline (Elavil) • Doxepin (Adapin) • Amoxapine (Asendin) • Maprotiline (Ludiomil)
Antiarrhythmics	• Quinidine • Procainamide • Disopyramide
Anticholinergics	• Atropine • Scopolamine hydrobromide • Clidinium bromide (Quarzan) • Glycopyrrolate (Robinul) • Mepenzolate bromide (Cantil) • Oxybutynin (Ditropan) • Flavoxate HCl (Urispas) • Hyoscyamine sulfate (Anaspaz) • Belladonna • Homatropine methylbromide • Propantheline bromide (Pro Banthine) • Dicyclomine HCl (Bentyl)
Anti-Parkinsonian agents	• Trihexyphenidyl HCl (Artane) • Benztropine Mesylate (Cogentin) • Amantadine HCl (Symmetrel) • Levodopa (Sinemet) • Bromocriptine Mesylate (Parlodel)
Hormonal agents	• Progesterone • Estrogen • Testosterone
Antipsychotics	• Haloperidol (Haldol) • Thiothixene (Navane) • Thioridazine (Mellaril) • Chlorpromazine (Thorazine) • Fluphenazine (Prolixin) • Prochlorperazine (Compazine)
Antihistamines	• Diphenhydramine HCl (Benadryl) • Chlorpheniramine (Chlor-Trimeton) • Brompheniramine (Dimetane) • Cyproheptadine (Periactin) • Hydroxyzine (Atarax, Vistaril)
Antihypertensives	• Hydralazine (Apresoline) • Nifedipine (Procardia)
Muscle relaxants	• Diazepam (Valium) • Baclofen (Lioresal) • Cyclobenzaprine (Flexeril)

(continued on next page)

Table 1 (continued)	
Miscellaneous	• Indomethacin (Indocin) • Carbamazepine (Tegretol) • Amphetamines • Dopamine • Vincristine • Morphine and other opioids • Anesthetic agents

patients if they wear pads or panty liners for protection, and what type they wear. Providers need to document how many pads they use in a 24-hour period and how damp the pads are when they are removed. If the patient does not endorse pad usage, providers can document how often patients need to change their undergarments and clothes. Pad weight testing can be done if the provider feels it is appropriate to quantify the amount of urine leaked over a 24-hour period, but this is usually reserved for research studies because of the burden on patients to save their pads and bring them to their appointment to be weighed.

A thorough medical and surgical history is important for the care of any patient. In the diagnosis of incontinence, it is critical to understand the number of pregnancies and live births a patient has had, if the deliveries were vaginal or cesarean section, the size of the infants, and if there was an episiotomy or other trauma during delivery. It is also appropriate to ask about any prior pelvic surgeries including hysterectomy and any previous incontinence procedures. Because of the frequency of concomitant procedures done for incontinence at the time of a hysterectomy, operative notes should be reviewed when available. Other surgeries that are important in the diagnosis of female urinary incontinence include spine surgeries and low pelvic surgeries for the colon. The practitioner should discuss with the patient if she is postmenopausal and, if so, for how long. It should be noted if the patient is on any type of hormones whether systemic or vaginal. To complete a review of systems, you must assess the patient's bowel function and see if there is any history of constipation or fecal incontinence. Because many procedures for incontinence may create scarring in the vagina, it is important to document if the patient is sexually active or plans to be in the future.

There are many comorbid conditions and medications that make incontinence more difficult to manage such as congestive heart failure and hypertension requiring the use of diuretics and uncontrolled diabetes mellitus. The patient's medications, laboratory values, and overall health should be examined in more detail.

Although this history may seem cumbersome, it is vitally important to find out the current characteristics of the patient's bathroom habits and how bothered they are by urgency or stress components of their incontinence. There are many useful validated survey tools that can make this process seem easier to accomplish during the usual time allotted during a new patient visit. These surveys can also follow the patient's symptoms over time, after treatment, to document improvement, as patients are not always reliable when asked if they have seen improvement.

PHYSICAL EXAMINATION OF THE INCONTINENT PATIENT

The components of a thorough physical examination of a woman with incontinence includes a general evaluation, an abdominal examination, a brief neurologic examination, and a detailed pelvic examination. The general evaluation should include the patient's general ability to understand the urge to urinate and the ability to get to the toilet in an appropriate amount of time. This can be accomplished by asking the patient the detailed questions in your history and also by asking the patient to get up from a chair and move to the examination table to prepare for the evaluation.

The abdominal examination should take into account the patient's abdominal girth, assess for any hernias, any pain to palpation of the bladder or any abdominal quadrants, and any previous surgical scars from hysterectomy, cholecystectomy, appendectomy, or others. The neurologic examination should generally determine if the patient has equal sensation of bilateral lower limbs or anything that would make the use of incontinence devices difficult (ie, contractures from previous cerebrovascular accident, blindness, or other impairments that would make things such as pessary placement or clean intermittent catheterization difficult).

The pelvic examination of the incontinent patient begins with a thorough investigation of the skin. It is important to evaluate for skin changes from chronic pad use and dampness. These changes could represent a contact dermatitis, candidiasis, lichen sclerosis, or even vulvar cancer. After this has been evaluated, the external labia can be gently spread manually and the vaginal mucosa can be evaluated. After the labia majora are spread, the practitioner should evaluate the urethral meatus for location, relative size, and the appearance of any urethral caruncle or prolapse. This is also the time to evaluate the vaginal mucosa for any atrophy. Vaginal atrophy is characterized as inflammation and thinning of the vaginal mucosa and gives the appearance of a light pink to pale white mucosa. In severe cases, there can be petechiae present.[9]

After the meatus and mucosa have been inspected, the hemi speculum should be inserted toward the vaginal apex on the posterior vaginal wall and gentle downward pressure applied. The patient can then be asked to Valsalva, and the anterior vaginal wall can be evaluated for the appearance of a cystocele. It should also be noted if the patient has any leakage from the urethra during Valsalva, and if not, the patient can be asked to give a strong cough to assist in the documentation of stress urinary incontinence. After evaluating for any cystocele, the hemi speculum can be withdrawn and reinserted along the anterior vaginal wall with gentle upward pressure. The patient should then be asked again to give a strong cough or Valsalva, and the presence of a rectocele should be observed. Finally, the speculum can be removed and discarded and manual examination can begin. The manual examination for incontinence should include palpation under the urethra for any bulge that could represent a urethral diverticulum and for the position of the vaginal apex or cervix. It is appropriate at this time to ask the patient to perform a Kegel muscle squeeze. This allows the provider to assess the strength of the patient's pelvic floor and also to see if the patient knows how to perform a proper Kegel contraction. The Kegel contraction should be firm around 1 finger inserted into the vagina while the abdominal and thigh muscles remain relaxed.

Regarding documentation of the female pelvic examination, since 1996 the Pelvic Organ Prolapse Quantification system (POP-Q) is the staging documentation most used in a research setting. This system was created to provide objective measurement among multiple examiners. The POP-Q system, a series of 9 specific points are measured with relationship to the hymenal ring. The points proximal to the ring are negative and the points distal to the ring are positive. The genital hiatus represents the size of the vaginal opening, and the perineal body refers to the distance between the vagina and the anus. The total vaginal length is measured by reducing the prolapse and measuring the depth of the vagina (**Table 2**).[10]

Table 2	
Pelvic organ prolapse quantification measurement sites	
Point	Description
Aa	Anterior vaginal wall 3 cm proximal to the hymen
Ba	Most distal position of anterior vaginal wall
C	Cervix
D	Posterior fornix (omit is hysterectomy)
Ap	Posterior vaginal wall 3 cm proximal to hymen
Bp	Most distal portion of posterior vaginal wall
Tvl	Depth of vagina when any prolapse is reduced

Data from Bump RC, Mattiasson A, Bø K, et al. The standardization of terminology of female pelvic organ prolapse and pelvic floor dysfunction. Am J Obstet Gynecol 1996;175(1):10–7.

DIAGNOSTIC STUDIES IN THE INCONTINENT FEMALE

In straightforward cases of female urinary incontinence, minimal diagnostic studies are indicated. These studies should aim toward diagnosing the reversible and more complex cases of urinary incontinence and include a urinalysis and postvoid residual (PVR). The urinalysis will reveal if the patient has any leukocytes or nitrites in her urine, and, if so, it should be sent for culture and any infection treated appropriately. It will also show if there is excessive protein in the urine, which should be referred to the nephrology department. Glucose in the urine could signal poorly controlled diabetes that can exacerbate urinary frequency and should be referred to the patient's primary care provider or endocrinologist. Finally, hematuria can be assessed and, if present, will need to be evaluated to ensure that the patient does not have an underlying urologic malignancy.

The PVR is a very simple, but critical, test in the diagnosis of female incontinence. It can be obtained with either a bladder scanner in the clinic or an "in-and-out" catheter after the patient has voided if a bladder scanner is not available or the patient's body habitus makes the bladder scanner unreliable. There is not a clearly defined acceptable value for a PVR. In general terms, a PVR of less than 50 is considered normal. Higher PVRs are acceptable if you know the patient's bladder capacity and feel confident that they are emptying more than half to two-thirds of that capacity.[11] It is important to understand how well the patient empties the bladder both to ensure that the patient does not have a more complex urologic condition and also because most treatments for urinary incontinence can cause the adverse reaction of urinary retention, and care needs to be taken in patients who empty poorly at baseline evaluation. It is also important to be sure that the patient is not in overflow incontinence, which is a serious condition that can cause increased pressure to the kidneys and lead to kidney failure. If the patient has a high PVR, then placement of a Foley catheter, documentation of creatinine level, and monitoring for post–obstructive diuresis should be considered.

In cases in which the patient's medical history, previous surgeries, physical examination, or diagnostic testing cause concern for a more complicated diagnosis, there are several tests that can be used. These include urodynamics (UDS) with or without video, voiding cystourethrogram (VCUG), and cystoscopy.

Urodynamics is a study that documents the capacity of the bladder, looks for any changes in compliance during filling, tries to elicit any incontinence with cough and Valsalva at increasing levels of fluid in the bladder, and measures the force of detrusor contraction and uroflow during voiding. This study is also able to document the post-void residual. This study involves a small catheter placed into the bladder and filled slowly with water. The patient is asked to report to the technician when they have first sensation that there is fluid in the bladder (under 100 mL is considered normal). They are also asked to report any sensation of urgency and when their bladder is at maximum capacity. Once at maximum capacity, the patient is given permission to void and the catheter, remaining in the bladder, records the detrusor contraction while the uroflow machine records the maximum force, the duration, and the average force of the urine stream. There is additionally a catheter in the rectum or vagina that records the abdominal pressure and documents if the patient is straining during voiding. Finally, there is a needle or patch for electromyogram recording of the pelvic floor that can document dyssynergia during voiding. This study can also be done with fluoroscopy for visualization of the urinary sphincter, documentation of reflux, presence of bladder or urethral diverticula, and other abnormalities. In general, only patients who can tell the technician when they have first sensation and can try to void on command should be referred for urodynamic testing.

If video urodynamics are not available, or not the preferred choice of study, a VCUG can be used to visualize the bladder and urethra. Although there are many protocols for cystograms, the best one for assessing urinary incontinence is the following. During the VCUG, a catheter is placed into the bladder and the bladder is instilled with a radiopaque fluid until the patient states that her bladder is full. The patient should be standing during this study so that gravity can exert force on the patient and they can then cough and Valsalva to assess for stress incontinence around the Foley catheter and the presence of a cystocele. The catheter can then be removed and the patient can again cough and Valsalva. Finally, the patient can be instructed to void and, if the patient is standing and lateral films are obtained, the urethra can be assessed for various abnormalities including meatal stenosis, urethral diverticulum, and how well the patient empties.

Although cystoscopy is rarely indicated in the evaluation of uncomplicated female incontinence, it is often necessary when initial urinalysis finds microscopic hematuria. It can also be useful when the practitioner suspects stress incontinence, but no leakage has been elicited on physical examination. In this situation, the bladder should be evaluated in the usual fashion, and when the surveillance of the urothelium is completed, the bladder can be filled with sterile water until the patient notes that the bladder is full. The scope can be slowly withdrawn, paying attention to the location of the sphincter muscle. After the cystoscope has been withdrawn, the patient can be asked to give a strong cough with particular attention given to leakage per urethra. If the patient still fails to demonstrate incontinence, the patient can be asked to do a standing stress test.

It should also be noted that in the complicated incontinence diagnosis, the patient may require all of these tests to document the mechanism of their incontinence, confirm that there are no foreign bodies in the vagina or bladder, and ensure that there is no evidence of obstruction from prior procedures or strictures.

TREATMENT OF FEMALE INCONTINENCE

Once the correct mechanism of leakage is confirmed, the patient can be offered appropriate treatment. Treatment should proceed in a stepwise pattern from least invasive to most invasive. It should also be noted that treatment of the incontinent patient should only occur or progress when the patient is dissatisfied and desires a better quality of life. If a patient is not bothered by her incontinence, or is not bothered enough to proceed with surgical intervention, then that patient should be allowed to delay or refuse treatment.

Stress Urinary Incontinence

The treatment of uncomplicated stress incontinence starts with lifestyle changes. These changes can include weight loss, fluid restriction, timed voiding, Kegel muscle training, and biofeedback. There is also a subset of incontinence devices that can be used. Fluid restriction should be modest and kept to 64 ounces per day of total fluid. If nocturia is a patient complaint, the patient can be asked to stop fluids 2 to 3 hours before bedtime.[12] The principle behind timed voiding in the treatment of stress incontinence is to prevent the bladder from becoming too full. If we know that a patient will leak urine if it has been more than 4 hours since they last voided, the goal with timed voiding should be to void every 3 hours based on the clock, rather than on sensation of bladder fullness.

Kegel exercises, and more broadly, pelvic floor physical therapy, are excellent tools in the treatment of stress urinary incontinence. Some basic pelvic floor exercises can be described to the patient at the time of her appointment including the proper way to do a Kegel squeeze: contract the muscles used to prevent the flow of urine or prevent flatus, keep stomach and thighs relaxed, number of times per day, and repetitions per time. However, if these measures are unsuccessful or the patient seems to need more hands-on instruction, a pelvic floor physical therapist can be invaluable. This therapy can be done by a trained patient care professional in an office setting or by a physical therapist with advanced training in pelvic floor conditions.[13]

The use of incontinence devices in women with stress incontinence is underutilized. These devices act as a mechanism of resistance for the involuntary loss of urine and to restore the proper position of the urethra. They include incontinence pessaries, which are fitted by a trained professional and reside high in the vagina. There is typically a knob or some other structure that provides increased pressure on the posterior aspect of the urethra and helps to prevent leakage. A well fitted pessary should not be felt by the patient and can be removed if it interferes with intercourse. Women can be taught how to remove, clean, and reinsert the pessary and based on their comfort level, can remove it nightly, weekly, or monthly. It is advised that in postmenopausal women, vaginal hormone replacement therapy is used to prevent ulceration of the vaginal mucosa by the pessary. There is also an over-the-counter option for women for the treatment of stress incontinence. This device, called the Impressa by Poise, is inserted into the vagina and deploys like a tampon to provide pressure on the posterior urethra and prevent stress incontinence. The device can be worn for up to 12 hours at a time and could be useful in patients with daytime or exercise-induced SUI.

Once conservative measures fail, the treatment of uncomplicated stress incontinence is based on procedures. There is no role for oral medication or botulinum toxin (Botox) in the treatment of stress incontinence. The treatments include urethral bulking agents and sling procedures.

Urethral bulking agents have a long history starting with C collagen injection in 1993 until 2011. More recently, materials such as Durasphere, Macroplastique, and Coaptite have been used all with similar efficacy. These procedures can be done with the patient awake in the clinic or in a sedated outpatient surgery setting. A rigid cystoscope is inserted into the urethra, and the external sphincter muscle is visualized. Then the bulking agent of choice is injected into the sphincter muscle until coaptation is observed. The cystoscope is then withdrawn, and the patient can be sent home. Complications are rare and include sterile abscess formation, erosion or migration of the injected material, and urethral prolapse. Reinjection is often required, and results are less effective than a sling surgery procedure, but patients may opt for this procedure if they are not good surgical candidates, if they are not bothered enough to go through a more aggressive surgery and recovery, or as an adjunct treatment when they still have incontinence after the placement of a midurethral sling.[14]

If urethral bulking agents fail, or the patient is not interested in trying them, a sling procedure should be considered. There are many sling products that are used today, and a sling can also be made with the patient's native fascia. Midurethral slings are an effective treatment of stress urinary incontinence.[15] Each type of midurethral sling, whether made with fascia or mesh, has specific complications that the patient needs to be extensively counseled about before the surgical procedure. These can include urinary retention, dyspareunia, erosion of the synthetic product into the vagina or urinary system, recurrent urinary tract infections, and others. Several other surgical procedures for urinary incontinence are available and may be appropriate for patients based on their degree of pelvic organ prolapse, need for a concomitant hysterectomy, and other factors.

Urgency Incontinence

Urgency incontinence, like stress incontinence, should proceed in a stepwise fashion from least invasive to most invasive and should start with lifestyle management. Although patients suffering with urgency incontinence will benefit from fluid restriction and timed voiding, they will also likely benefit from avoidance of bladder irritants and bladder training. Bladder training can often be combined with pelvic floor muscle therapy and involves timed voiding and suppression of urges through relaxation and distraction techniques. Over time, the intervals of the voiding can be gradually increased. A voiding diary is especially helpful to monitor compliance and progress in these patients. Diaries are also helpful in patients trying to eliminate bladder irritants. There are several lists available, and they are long, but if patients try to avoid spicy foods, acidic foods, alcohol, coffee, tea, carbonation, and artificial sweeteners for 2 weeks and see a benefit, they may be able to improve their urgency symptoms by avoiding these in the future.

If lifestyle modification is not effective in treating urgency incontinence, the next line of treatment is medical management. Oxytbutynin has been available for the longest, time and it exists in several forms: an immediate release, an extended-release formulation (oxybutynin XL), and topical formulations that are available over the counter in a daily patch (Oxytrol) or a gel that can be applied daily. An additional 6 medications in the same drug class have been released since oxybutynin first hit the market. These drugs are classified as anticholinergics or antimuscarinics and act by blocking the anticholinergic receptor on smooth muscle. Although these medications try to target the M3 receptor on the bladder specifically, they also have some affinity for the other M1-M5 receptors. Because of this finding, they all carry the side-effect profile of dry eyes, dry mouth, constipation, and urinary retention. Furthermore, the older anticholinergics need to be given with caution in the elderly because of crossing the blood-brain barrier, which can lead to confusion (**Table 3**).

Finally, in 2015, a new drug was approved in the United States for the treatment of urgency urinary incontinence and OAB. This drug, mirabegron, is a selective β-3 agonist, and because it binds to a different receptor, the side effects are much different and include a modest increase in blood pressure, headache, and urinary retention. It can be used as a first-line drug treatment for urgency incontinence or in combination with an anticholinergic.

When medication does adequately control urgency incontinence and OAB, or the patient does not tolerate the side effects of medications, treatment options for

Table 3
Antimuscarinic agents used in the management of overactive bladder

Drug Name		Starting Doses	Generic Availability
Darifenacin	Extended-release oral (Enablex)	7.5-mg PO daily	No
Fesoterodine	Extended-release oral (Toviaz)	4-mg PO daily	No
Oxybutynin	Immediate-release oral (Ditropan)	5-mg PO BID-TID	Yes
	Extended-release oral (Ditropan XL)	5-mg PO daily	
	Transdermal gel (Gelnique)	Apply 1 package topically daily	No
	Transdermal patch (Oxytrol)	Apply one 3.9-mg/24-h patch every 3–4 d	
Solifenacin	Immediate-release oral (Vesicare)	5-mg PO daily	No
Tolterodine	Immediate-release oral (Detrol)	2-mg PO BID	No
	Extended-release oral (Detrol LA)	4-mg PO daily	
Trospium	Immediate-release oral (Sanctura)	20-mg PO BID	Yes
	Extended-release oral (Sanctura XR)	60-mg PO QAM	No

Abbreviations: BID, twice a day; OAB, overactive bladder; PO, by mouth; QAM, every morning; TID, 3 times a day.

From Bridgeman MB, Taft C. Overactive Bladder Management: Challenges and Opportunities. Pharmacy Times. Available at: https://www.pharmacytimes.org/landing/276. Accessed August 21, 2017; with permission.

refractory OAB can be offered. These treatments include percutaneous tibial nerve stimulation (PTNS), onabotulinum toxin A (Botox), and sacral neuromodulation.

PTNS is a procedure in which a health care provider inserts a 28-gauge needle near the posterior tibial nerve by finding the landmark of the medial malleolus and finding a spot about 2 fingerbreadths superior and 1 fingerbreadth posterior to that area. This small needle is then attached to an electric current, and the machine is turned up to a tolerable level for the patient. Classically, the patient will feel the sensation toward the ball of the foot, and not around the needle, and the great toe will dorsiflex. Treatments take 30 minutes per session, and the patient is expected to complete weekly sessions for 12 weeks. Small studies have shown that PTNS is more effective than no treatment or drug treatment.[16]

The injection of onabotulinum toxin A (Botox), has been approved by the US Food and Drug Administration for the treatment of neurogenic OAB since 2011 and idiopathic OAB since 2012. To administer this agent, the patient has lidocaine solution instilled into the bladder for a few minutes followed by insertion of a rigid or flexible cystoscope. The bladder is inspected and the ureteral orifices are noted as they should be avoided. Then, if the patient has neurogenic OAB or idiopathic OAB the patient receives injections into the bladder mucosa of 200 units or 100 units, respectively. The scope is withdrawn and the patient is sent home. This can be done in the office or outpatient surgical setting. Care should be taken to ensure the patient does not have an active urinary tract infection at the time of Botox injection, and the patient should be counseled about the risk of urinary retention happening in about 20% of injections for neurogenic diagnoses and 5% of injections for idiopathic diagnoses. It is wise, therefore, not to inject Botox unless the patient is willing to learn clean intermittent catheterization should there be a problem with urinary retention. Average length of time for Botox effectiveness varies but is around 6 to 9 months.

Sacral neuromodulation is similar to the principle of PTNS; however, this treatment more accurately targets the S3 afferent nerve in the lower spine. The patient must be neurologically intact at this level to benefit from this procedure. It is typically started with a trial that can be performed in the clinic or in the operating room, and if the patient has improvement in her symptoms over the next 1 to 2 weeks, then a permanent device is implanted. Patients can be instructed in how to turn on and off their device when needed and can alter their stimulation program if the benefits decrease over time. The expected battery life is typically 8 to 12 years for this device, so younger patients may need additional surgeries over time. It is also currently contraindicated to have a pelvic MRI with the Interstim (Medtronic, Minneapolis, USA) device in place, so patients with chronic conditions requiring MRI for surveillance may not be appropriate candidates for this treatment for refractory urgency incontinence.

Since the development of PTNS, Botox, and Interstim, it is rare that a more aggressive incontinence surgery needs to be performed for urgency incontinence, but in very severe cases, the patient can be offered an augmentation cystoplasty, in which the bladder is opened and a piece of bowel is added to the dome of the bladder. This surgery does have significant recovery, but has excellent results. However, long-term data suggest an increase in the need to do self-catheterization over time. There are also reports of urinary diversion for severe urinary urgency incontinence.

CHALLENGING INCONTINENCE PATIENTS

There are many types of incontinence, and the diagnosis is not always clear to the health care provider. Although diagnostic testing does exist, it is not a requirement before treatment, and many patients have surgery without ever having formal UDS. Even when a woman is referred for UDS, it may not reproduce her leakage, as the conditions in a urodynamic testing room do not exactly mimic real life. Not all women will have a successful result from any incontinence treatment or surgical procedure for incontinence. One woman may find surgery a success if she can decrease her pad usage by 75%, whereas another patient may badly want to be completely dry. Women who have had their incontinence treated and continue to leak are especially difficult to diagnose and treat. If a stress incontinence surgery is done too loosely, the patient may continue to leak. If it is done to tight, she may not be able to empty her bladder. There is also evidence that when the bladder is under pressure, it may become spastic and the patient may experience symptoms of urgency. Therefore, any new incontinence in a patient that has a history of prior incontinence surgery should be complicated. These patients require advanced testing, thorough reading of the prior operative reports, and consideration for referral to an experienced tertiary care facility who treat these patients often.

SUMMARY

Incontinence is very common, despite the fact it is not often discussed. Although it may not carry significant mortality, it does contribute to feelings of depression, anxiety, and social withdrawal. It is more common with aging and is very common in the nursing home population, often being the final diagnosis leading the caregiver to consider nursing home placement. It can be easy to diagnose by simply talking to patients about their bladder habits and asking if they have incontinence. When the patient history is straightforward and the physical examination supports a simple diagnosis of incontinence, there are good results with lifestyle modification of weight loss, fluid restriction, and pelvic floor muscle therapy. When conservative measures fail, medications for urgency incontinence and procedures for both stress and urge incontinence can be offered to patients. When cases are more complicated, there is advanced testing to reproduce the leakage and help the patients accordingly with assistance from centers of excellence around the country who specialize in these complicated cases. As the population lives longer and grows older, we are more likely, as health care professionals, to encounter more women who want treatment for their incontinence and do not see it as something to be expected with normal aging. We need to be prepared to ask about incontinence, listen to patient's concerns about their leakage, and have some tools to begin treatment.

REFERENCES

1. Harris SS. Care Seeking and treatment for urinary incontinence in a diverse population. J Urol 2007;177(2):680.
2. Hannestad YS. Help-seeking and associated factors in female urinary incontinence. The Norweigian EPINCONT Study. Epidemiology of incontinence in the county of Nord-Trondelag. Scand J Prim Health Care 2002;20(2):102–7.
3. Morrill M. Seeking healthcare for pelvic floor disorders: a population-based study. Am J Obstet Gynecol 2007;197(1):86.e1-6.
4. Offermans MP. Prevalence of urinary incontinence and associated risk factors in nursing home residents: a systematic review. Neurourol Urodyn 2009;28(4):288.
5. Rortveit G. Age and type-dependent effects of parity on urinary incontinence: the Norwegian EPINCONT study. Obstet Gynecol 2001;98(6):1004.
6. Coyne KS. The impact of overactive bladder, incontinence and other lower urinary tract symptoms on quality of life, work productivity, sexuality and emotional well-being in men and women: results from the EPIC study. BJU Int 2008;101(11): 1388.
7. Morrison A, Levy R. Fraction of nursing home admissions attributable to urinary incontinence. Value Health 2006;9(4):272.
8. Curtis LA, Dolan TS, Cespedes RD. Acute urinary retention and urinary incontinence. Emerg Med Clin North Am 2001;19:591.
9. Portman DJ, Gass ML. Vulvovaginal Atrophy Terminology Consensus Conference Panel Genitourinary syndrome of menopause: new terminology for vulvovaginal atrophy from the International Society for the Study of Women's Sexual Health and the North American Menopause Society. Menopause 2014;21(10):1063–8.
10. Kobashi KC. Campbell's urology. In: Wein A, Kavoussi L, Partin A, et al, editors. Evaluation and management of women with urinary incontinence and pelvic prolapse. Chapter 71. Philadelphia: W.B. Saunders; 2007. p. 1697–709.e3.
11. Nager CW. Reference urodynamic values for stress incontinent women. Neurourol Urodyn 2007;26(3):333–40.
12. Dallosso HM. The association of diet and other lifestyle factors with overactive bladder and stress incontinence: a longitudinal study in women. BJU Int 2003; 92(1):69–77.
13. Dumoulin C, Hay-Smith EJC, Mac Habée-Séguin G. Pelvic floor muscle training versus no treatment, or inactive control treatments, for urinary incontinence in women. Cochrane Database Syst Rev 2014;5:CD005654.

14. Kirchin V, Page T, Keegan PE, et al. Urethral injection therapy for urinary inconti-
    nence in women. Cochrane Database Syst Rev 2017;7:CD003881.
15. Rehman H, Bezerra CA, Bruschini H, et al. Traditional suburethral sling operations
    for urinary incontinence in women. Cochrane Database Syst Rev 2017;7:
    CD001754.
16. Gormley EA. Diagnosis and treatment of overactive bladder (non-neurogenic) in
    adults: AUA/SUFU guideline amendment. J Urol 2015;193(5):1572.

Male Lower Urinary Tract Symptoms

Todd J. Doran, EdD, PA-C

KEYWORDS

- Benign prostatic hypertrophy • Benign prostatic enlargement
- Lower urinary tract symptoms • Voiding dysfunction • Prostatic obstruction
- Bladder outlet obstruction • Bladder neck obstruction • Physician assistant

KEY POINTS

- Symptoms often correlate with the location of the problem and guide medication choices.
- Prostate-specific antigen is a good proxy for prostatic size and guides medication choices.
- Lower urinary tract symptoms and erectile dysfunction are often comorbid conditions and both should be assessed at the initial visit and at all follow-ups. Medication choices can positively and negatively affect each condition.
- Specialty referral should be reserved for patients who have been thoroughly evaluated and medical management initiated with adequate time to respond to therapy. Exceptions are those with an abnormal initial evaluation: abnormal laboratory tests, abnormal physical examinations, or high index of suspicion for urethral stricture disease.

INTRODUCTION

Lower urinary tract symptoms (LUTS) is a nonspecific term describing urinary symptoms that are classified as storage, voiding, or postmicturition symptoms as described by an international consensus conference.[1] The prevalence of male LUTS increases with age and negatively affects quality of life. Decompensation can present with acute urinary retention and renal failure and urinary incontinence, which is a leading cause of skilled nursing placement. LUTS and erectile dysfunction (ED) are comorbid conditions and should be assessed together at the initial visit and at follow-up visits.[2,3] The history, physical examination, and diagnostic studies are straightforward and medical therapy decisions should target the suspected cause (bladder vs outlet). Adequate time for response to therapy and medication titration are also important

Disclosures: The author has nothing to disclose.
Physician Associate Program, Department of Family and Preventive Medicine, The University of Oklahoma Health Sciences Center, College of Medicine, 940 Stanton L. Young Boulevard, Suite 357, Oklahoma City, OK 73104, USA
E-mail address: todd-doran@ouhsc.edu

Physician Assist Clin 3 (2018) 83–102
https://doi.org/10.1016/j.cpha.2017.08.012
2405-7991/18/© 2017 Elsevier Inc. All rights reserved.

physicianassistant.theclinics.com

considerations when determining whether the patient has failed medical therapy and warrants specialty referral.

EVALUATION OF LOWER URINARY TRACT SYMPTOMS
History

An adequate urologic history is easily obtained with standardized questionnaires, but it is common for primary care to inadequately obtain a voiding history, erectile function history, or ask about urinary incontinence. The utility of standardized patient questionnaires in obtaining urinary and erectile function helps to establish a baseline with which to compare the response to therapy, in addition to severity and patient bother. The American Urological Association Symptom Index (AUASI) is the most widely used tool to obtain a urologic history (**Table 1**).[4] The International Prostate Symptom Score (IPSS) adds an eighth question referring to the patient's perceived quality of life: "If you were to spend the rest of your life with your urinary condition just the way it is now, how would you feel about that?" and this is scored from 0 to 6 with 0 meaning delighted and 6 meaning terrible. Symptom severity is extrapolated based on the total score for questions 1 to 7: less than 8 is mild, 8 to 19 moderate, and greater than 19 is severe. Mild symptoms with normal examination are usually managed conservatively without medication.

Table 2 categorizes symptoms into storage, voiding, and postmicturition, which typically correspond with source of the problem: storage corresponds with bladder; voiding from bladder neck to meatus; and postmicturition can be mixed or other.[1] Predominant significant nocturia is defined as awakened 2 or more times per night to void. These patients should complete a frequency volume chart for 2 to 3 days. The frequency volume chart shows 24-hour polyuria or nocturnal polyuria when present,

---

Table 1
American Urological Association symptom score

1. Over the past month, how often have you had a sensation of not emptying your bladder completely after you finished urinating?
2. Over the past month, how often have you had to urinate again <2 h after you finished urinating?
3. Over the past month, how often have you found that you stopped and started again several times when you urinated?
4. Over the past month, how often have you found it difficult to postpone urination?
5. Over the past month, how often have you had a weak urinary stream?
6. Over the past month, how often have you had to push or strain to begin urination?
7. Over the past month, how many times did you most typically get up to urinate from the time you went to bed at night until the time you got up in the morning?

Scoring for questions 1–6
   0 Indicates not at all; 1 indicates <1 in 5; 2 indicates less than half the time; 3 indicates about half the time; 4 indicates more than half the time; 5 indicates almost always.

Scoring for question 7
   The number corresponds with the number of times you got up to urinate after going to bed for the night and the maximum score of 5 means you got up 5 times or more.

Interpretation	
Score	Severity
0–7	Mild
8–19	Moderate
20–35	Severe

Table 2 Urinary symptoms		
Storage	**Voiding**	**Postmicturition**
Urgency	Slow stream	Incomplete emptying
Daytime frequency	Intermittent stream	Postvoid dribble
Nocturia	Hesitancy	
Urge incontinence	Straining to void	
	Dysuria	
	Terminal dribble	

the first of which has been defined as greater than 3 L of total output over 24 hours.[5] Patients with bothersome symptoms are advised to aim for a urine output of 1 L/24 h. Nocturnal polyuria is diagnosed when more than 33% of the 24-hour urine output occurs at night and typically has a systemic physiologic cause, and optimally managing the systemic cause may improve the symptoms.[5]

The International Index of Erectile Function (IIEF) is the most commonly used validated standardized patient questionnaire to assess erectile function.[6] The full questionnaire is a 15-question inventory; however, the most clinically used is the 5-question version. Prevalence and severity of ED and LUTS are similar and reports in the general male population show that 13% to 29% had moderate to severe LUTS assessed by AUASI and 8% to 35% had moderate to severe ED assessed by IIEF.[6] Overall prevalence of comorbid LUTS and ED of any severity was 71% to 80% for those men seeking treatment of their LUTS.[6] The clinical relevance is that both conditions must be evaluated at the time of presentation and can drive treatment decisions as well as reassessment on follow-up because of the side effects of some medications used to treat LUTS, particularly 5-alpha reductase inhibitors (5ARI). Further discussion regarding the evaluation and treatment of ED is covered in Patrick Dougherty's article, "Erectile Dysfunction," in this issue.

Further pertinent urologic history related to LUTS is directed to the lower urinary tract. History of urinary tract infections (UTIs), hematuria, urinary retention, presence and type of urinary incontinence, sexually transmitted infections (especially gonorrhea, even remotely), urethral instrumentation (catheter, cystoscopy), prostate-related surgery, perineal trauma, pelvic fracture, and discussion of stool patterns (constipation, incontinence) are applicable when assessing LUTS. This history guides the physical examination, laboratory testing, and special testing to narrow the differential diagnosis.

Physical Examination

The physical examination should evaluate potential sources for the patient's LUTS and help to narrow the differential diagnosis. Examination of the phallus should include foreskin mobility, meatus size and position, surgical scars, rectal tone, and prostate size and symmetry, and inspection of the sacrum to look for external signs for spinae bifida (hairy patch, dimple, dark spot, lumbar swelling). Prostate size is critical to determine whether treatment with 5ARI is indicated.[5,7,8] Clinical trials have shown the relationship between prostate-specific antigen (PSA) total level and prostate size.[7,8] Enlarged prostate is defined as (>30 cm³) or a PSA total level of greater than or equal to 1.6 ng/mL.[7,8] Men with enlarged prostates are correlated with moderate to severe LUTS, acute urinary retention, urinary incontinence, and UTI.[7]

Laboratory Testing

Urinalysis (UA) and PSA testing are reasonable screening laboratory tests. UA can assess for evidence of infection and presence of hematuria. Urine microscopy is performed for positive dipstick results. Urine culture is reserved for patients with UA evidence of infection (nitrite positive, leukocyte esterase positive, and heme positive). Hematuria evaluation is covered in Priyanka Tilak and colleagues' article, "Evaluation and Work-up of Hematuria in Adults," in this issue. PSA testing can be used as a proxy to estimate prostate size and to screen for prostate cancer in susceptible populations.[5] PSA interpretation and evaluation is covered in Ryan Lewis' article, "Prostate Cancer Screening," in this issue. The American Urological Association (AUA) recommends against the routine measurement of serum creatinine levels in the initial evaluation of men with LUTS.[5] It is reasonable to assess serum creatinine level if it is an important consideration in medication selection.

Special Testing

AUA clinical guidelines advise that all testing, including uroflowmetry, postvoid residual (PVR), pressure-flow urodynamics, and cystoscopy, is considered optional. The Sixth International Consultation on New Developments in Prostate Cancer and Prostate Diseases recommends urine flow rate measurement (Q_{max}) and PVR at baseline and follow-up.[1] PVR can be measured by ultrasonography or in-and-out catheterization. PVR of 300 mL usually warrants specialty referral. **Fig. 1** shows a normal uroflow

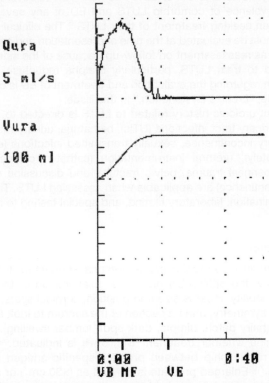

Fig. 1. Normal shape uroflow. Normal bell-shaped curve. Q_{max} of 25 mL/s and a voiding time of approximately 18 seconds with an estimated voided volume of 450 mL. PVR of 25 mL, and this must be obtained via bladder scan, ultrasonography, or catheter.

and **Fig. 2** shows a classic flattened pattern caused by obstruction (urethral stricture, prostate, or bladder neck). Bladder outlet obstruction can be accurately diagnosed in men with a Q_{max} less than 10 mL/s and an AUASI greater than 16.[9]

TREATMENT

Management decisions are based on symptoms (storage vs voiding), laboratory testing, special testing, and prostate volume.[5,7,8] Alpha-adrenergic receptor antagonists (α-blockers) are first-line choices for LUTS with predominantly voiding symptoms. Terazosin (Hytrin), doxazosin (Cardura), tamsulosin (Flomax), alfuzosin (Uroxatral), and silodosin (Rapaflo) are all equally efficacious, but terazosin and doxazosin must be titrated (**Table 3**).[5] Patients should be warned about the risk of retrograde ejaculation, which can be troubling to patients, especially those who are actively pursuing fertility. Intraoperative floppy iris syndrome is associated with tamsulosin (Flomax) in particular, but the risk is known with all α-blockers.[5] Initiation of α-blocker therapy should be avoided in men until cataract surgery has been completed, and there should be disclosure of α-blocker exposure to the ophthalmologist for all others with no planned cataract surgery.[5] Reassessment should take place once a maximum dose has been achieved for at least 1 month.

Combination therapy with a 5ARI (**Table 4**) should be reserved for those men with an enlarged prostate described on digital rectal examination or a PSA value greater than or equal to 1.6 ng/mL.[7,8] Clinical trials with combination therapy have been with finasteride (Proscar) plus doxazosin (Cardura) or dutasteride (Avodart) plus tamsulosin (Flomax).[7,8] Both studies showed that PSA level was reduced by half within 6 months and resulted in

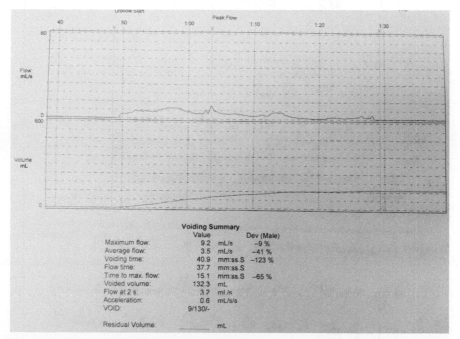

	Voiding Summary		
	Value		Dev (Male)
Maximum flow:	9.2	mL/s	−9 %
Average flow:	3.5	mL/s	−41 %
Voiding time:	40.9	mm:ss.S	−123 %
Flow time:	37.7	mm:ss.S	
Time to max. flow:	15.1	mm:ss.S	−65 %
Voided volume:	132.3	mL	
Flow at 2 s:	3.2	ml /s	
Acceleration:	0.6	mL/s/s	
VOID:	9/130/-		
Residual Volume:	_____	mL	

Fig. 2. Abnormal uroflow. Classic prolonged flattened curve. Q_{max} of 9.2 mL/s and a voiding time of approximately 41 seconds with an estimated voided volume of 132 mL. PVR of 150 mL, and this must be obtained via bladder scan, ultrasonography, or catheter.

Table 3
Alpha-adrenergic receptor antagonists

Medication	Dosage	Adverse Reactions	Renal Dosing
Terazosin (Hytrin)	1, 2, 5, and 10 mg. Maximum dosing is 20 mg Titration necessary over period of time to lessen orthostatic hypotension risk	>10%: Central nervous system: dizziness (9%–19%), myasthenia (7%–11%) 1%–10%: Cardiovascular: peripheral edema (1%–6%), orthostatic hypotension (1%–4%), palpitations (≤4%), tachycardia (≤2%), syncope (≤1%) Central nervous system: drowsiness (4%–5%), paresthesia (≤3%), vertigo (1%) Endocrine and metabolic: decreased libido (≤1%), weight gain (≤1%) Gastrointestinal: nausea (2%–4%) Genitourinary: impotence (≤2%) Neuromuscular and skeletal: limb pain (≤4%), back pain (≤2%) Ophthalmic: blurred vision (≤2%) Respiratory: nasal congestion (2%–6%), dyspnea (2%–3%), sinusitis (≤3%)	No dosage adjustment necessary

| Doxazosin (Cardura, Cardura XL) | 1, 2, 4, and 8 mg immediate release
4 and 8 mg extended release
Maximum dosing of 8 mg for either
formulation. Titration necessary
with immediate release formulation
over period of time to lessen
orthostatic hypotension risk | >10%:
Central nervous system: dizziness
(5%–19%), malaise (≤12%),
fatigue (8% to ≤12%), headache
(6%–10%)

1%–10%:
Cardiovascular: edema (3%–4%),
hypotension (1%–2%),
orthostatic hypotension (<1%–
2%), cardiac arrhythmia (1%),
facial edema (1%), flushing (1%),
palpitations (1%)
Central nervous system: drowsiness
(1%–5%), vertigo (2%–4%), pain
(2%), anxiety (1%), ataxia (1%),
hypertonia (1%), insomnia (1%),
movement disorder (1%),
myasthenia (1%)
Endocrine and metabolic: sexual
disorder (2%)
Gastrointestinal: abdominal pain
(2%), nausea (1%–2%), dyspepsia
(1%), xerostomia (1%)
Genitourinary: urinary incontinence
(1%), UTI (1%)
Neuromuscular and skeletal:
weakness (4%–7%), muscle
cramps (1%), myalgia (1%),
arthralgia (≤1%), arthritis (≤1%)
Ophthalmic: visual disturbance
(2%)
Otic: tinnitus (1%)
Renal: polyuria (2%)
Respiratory: respiratory tract
infection (5%), rhinitis (3%),
dyspnea (1%–3%), epistaxis (1%) | There are no dosage adjustments
provided in the manufacturer's
labeling |

(continued on next page)

Table 3
(continued)

Medication	Dosage	Adverse Reactions	Renal Dosing
Tamsulosin (Flomax)	0.04 mg Maximum dosing 0.08 mg	>10%: Cardiovascular: orthostatic hypotension (first dose: 6%–19%; symptomatic orthostatic hypotension [chronic therapy] 1%) Central nervous system: headache (19%–21%), dizziness (15%–17%) Genitourinary: ejaculation failure (8%–18%) Infection: infection (9%–11%) Respiratory: rhinitis (13%–18%) 1%–10%: Central nervous system: drowsiness (3%–4%), insomnia (1%–2%), vertigo (≤1%) Endocrine and metabolic: loss of libido (2%) Gastrointestinal: diarrhea (6%), nausea (4%) Neuromuscular and skeletal: weakness (8%–9%), back pain (7%–8%) Ophthalmic: blurred vision (≤2%) Respiratory: pharyngitis (6%), cough (3%–5%), sinusitis (4%)	CrCl ≥10 mL/min: no dosage adjustment necessary CrCl <10 mL/min: there are no dosage adjustments provided in the manufacturer's labeling (has not been studied)

Alfuzosin (Uroxatral)	10 mg	1%–10%: Central nervous system: dizziness (6%), fatigue (3%), headache (3%), pain (1%–2%) Gastrointestinal: abdominal pain (1%–2%), constipation (1%–2%), dyspepsia (1%–2%), nausea (1%–2%) Genitourinary: impotence (1%–2%) Respiratory: upper respiratory tract infection (3%), bronchitis (1%–2%), pharyngitis (1%–2%), sinusitis (1%–2%)	No dosage adjustments provided in the manufacturer's labeling; use with caution in severe renal impairment (CrCl <30 mL/min)
Silodosin (Rapaflo)	4 and 8 mg	>10%: Genitourinary: retrograde ejaculation (28%) 1%–10%: Cardiovascular: orthostatic hypotension (3%; increased in elderly ≥65 y up to 5%) Central nervous system: dizziness (3%), headache (2%), insomnia (1%–2%) Gastrointestinal: diarrhea (3%), abdominal pain (1%–2%) Genitourinary: PSA level increased (1%–2%) Neuromuscular and skeletal: weakness (1%–2%) Respiratory: nasal congestion (2%), rhinorrhea (1%–2%), sinusitis (1%–2%)	CrCl >50 mL/min: no dosage adjustment necessary CrCl 30–50 mL/min: 4 mg once daily CrCl <30 mL/min: use is contraindicated

Abbreviation: CrCl, creatinine clearance.
Data from Lexi-Comp. Drug Information Handbook: A Clinically Relevant Resource for All Healthcare Professionals. 26th edition. Hudson (OH): Wolters Kluwer; 2017.

Table 4
5-Alpha reductase inhibitors

Medication	Dosage	Adverse Reactions	Renal Dosing
Finasteride (Proscar)	1 and 5 mg. Use 5-mg dose for LUTS	>10%: Cardiovascular: orthostatic hypotension (combination therapy 18%; monotherapy 9%) Central nervous system: dizziness (combination therapy 23%; monotherapy 7%) Endocrine and metabolic: decreased libido (combination therapy 12%; monotherapy 2%–10%) Genitourinary: impotence (combination therapy 23%; monotherapy 5%–19%), ejaculatory disorder (combination therapy 14%; monotherapy <1%–7%) Neuromuscular and skeletal: weakness (combination therapy 17%; monotherapy 5%) 1%–10%: Cardiovascular: edema (combination therapy 3%; monotherapy 1%) Central nervous system: drowsiness (combination therapy 3%; monotherapy 2%) Dermatologic: skin rash (monotherapy 1%) Endocrine and metabolic: gynecomastia (monotherapy 1%–2%) Genitourinary: decreased ejaculate volume (monotherapy 2%–4%), breast tenderness (monotherapy ≤1%) Respiratory: dyspnea (combination therapy 2%; monotherapy 1%), rhinitis (combination therapy 2%; monotherapy 1%)	No dosage adjustment is necessary
Dutasteride (Avodart)	0.5 mg	1%–10%: Endocrine and metabolic: decreased libido (≤3%; incidence highest during first 6 mo of therapy), gynecomastia (including breast tenderness, breast enlargement; ≤1%), increased luteinizing hormone level, increased testosterone level, increased thyroid-stimulating hormone level Genitourinary: impotence (≤5%; incidence highest during first 6 mo of therapy), ejaculatory disorder (≤2%) Hematologic and oncologic: prostate cancer, high grade (≤1%)	No dosage adjustment is necessary

Data from Lexi-Comp. Drug Information Handbook: A Clinically Relevant Resource for All Healthcare Professionals. 26th edition. Hudson (OH): Wolters Kluwer; 2017.

decreased risk of acute urinary retention and the need for prostate-related surgery.[7,8] The reduction was nearly 80% and 67%, respectively, and the greatest risk reduction was observed the longer the patient was on combination therapy.[7,8] Combination therapy should not be initiated for less than 6 months with the intent that the patient will be on this therapy for years. Patients should be warned about the risk of gynecomastia, decreased libido, and ED. It can take many months to rebound after cessation of therapy.

Anticholinergics/antimuscarinics (**Table 5**) can be used as add-on therapy for incomplete symptom relief for patients on α-blockers. This class of medication can also be used as monotherapy for those patients with predominant storage symptoms. Consideration of which agent to start with depends on side effect profile, cost, drug interactions, renal dosing, and patient preference. Similar to α-blockers, anticholinergics/antimuscarinics can take up to 4 weeks on a steady state dosing to assess efficacy. Typical side effects are dry mouth, but can include confusion, especially in the elderly. Caution should be exercised for this class of medication for patients older than 65 years.[10–14] Historically, the risk of developing acute urinary retention is overstated; however, caution should be used in patients with severe voiding symptoms and those with increased PVRs. There is no consensus regarding the lower cutoff but a PVR less than 150 mL is reasonable and one of 250 to 300 mL is absolute.[5]

Miscellaneous agents (**Table 6**) such as tadalafil (Cialis) and mirabegron (Myrbetriq) are alternative agents to the other classes listed earlier. Tadalafil (Cialis) is the only phosphodiesterase-5 inhibitor (PDE5-I) that is US Food and Drug Administration (FDA) approved to treat comorbid LUTS and ED, and the typical dose is 5 mg daily. Concomitant use of α-blockers and PDE5-I requires caution. The advice is that one agent should be at a stable dose before adding the other class of medication. The clinical experience of this author is that α-blockers improve LUTS and ED better than PDE5-I, so initiation of an α-blocker followed by a PDE5-I makes clinical sense. Mirabegron (Myrbetriq) is a beta3-adrenoceptor agonist FDA approved to treat overactive bladder with less dry mouth and could be substituted for any of the anticholinergics/antimuscarinics listed in **Table 5**.

INDICATIONS FOR UROLOGIC REFERRAL

- Abnormal prostate examination
- Hematuria without evidence of infection
- Failure to respond to treatment
- Desire surgical treatment
- Men with persistent incontinence despite treatment
- PVRs greater than 300 mL or increasing in response to treatment
- Acute urinary retention
- Evidence of bilateral hydronephrosis

SURGICAL OPTIONS

There are several minimally invasive and surgical options for the treatment of LUTS.[5]

Minimally Invasive

- Transurethral needle ablation of the prostate
- Transurethral microwave thermotherapy

Surgical

- Transurethral holmium laser ablation of the prostate
- Transurethral holmium laser enucleation of the prostate

Table 5
Anticholinergics/antimuscarinics

Medication	Dosage	Adverse Reactions	Renal Dosing
Oxybutynin (Ditropan)	Immediate release: 5 mg 2–3 times daily; maximum, 5 mg 4 times daily Extended release: 5, 10 and 15 mg. Initial: 5–10 mg once daily, adjust dose in 5-mg increments at weekly intervals; maximum, 30 mg once daily Topical gel: apply contents of 1 sachet (100 mg/g) or 1 actuation of the pump (100 mg/g) once daily Transdermal: apply 1 3.9-mg/d patch twice weekly (every 3–4 d)	**>10%:** Central nervous system: dizziness (5%–17%), drowsiness (6%–14%) Gastrointestinal: xerostomia (35%–71%; dose related), constipation (9%–15%), nausea (5%–12%) **1%–10%:** Cardiovascular: cardiac arrhythmia (sinus; 1% to <5%), decreased blood pressure (1% to <5%), edema (1% to <5%), flushing (1% to <5%), hypertension (1% to <5%), palpitations (1% to <5%), peripheral edema (1% to <5%) Central nervous system: headache (8%), nervousness (7%), insomnia (3%–6%), confusion (1% to <5%), falling (1%–5%), fatigue (1% to <5%), flank pain (1% to <5%), pain (1% to <5%) Dermatologic: pruritus (1% to <5%), xeroderma (1% to <5%) Endocrine and metabolic: fluid retention (1% to <5%), hyperglycemia (1% to <5%), increased thirst (1% to <5%) Gastrointestinal: diarrhea (1%–8%), dyspepsia (5%–6%), abdominal pain (1% to <5%), dysphagia (1% to <5%), eructation (1% to <5%), flatulence (1% to <5%), unpleasant taste (1% to <5%), vomiting (1% to <5%), gastroesophageal reflux disease (≤1%) Genitourinary: urinary hesitancy (2%–9%), UTI (7%), urinary retention (1%–6%), cystitis (1% to <5%), dysuria (1% to <5%), pollakiuria (1% to <5%) Infection: fungal infection (1% to <5%) Neuromuscular and skeletal: arthralgia (1% to <5%), back pain (1% to <5%), limb pain (1% to <5%), weakness (1% to <5%) Ophthalmic: blurred vision (4%–10%), eye irritation (1% to <5%), keratoconjunctivitis sicca (1% to <5%), xerophthalmia (3%) Respiratory: asthma (1% to <5%), bronchitis (1% to <5%), cough (1% to <5%), dry throat (1% to <5%), hoarseness (1% to <5%), nasal congestion (1% to <5%), dry nose (1% to <5%), nasopharyngitis (1% to <5%), pharyngolaryngeal pain (1% to <5%), sinus congestion (1% to <5%), upper respiratory tract infection (1% to <5%)	No dosage adjustments provided in the manufacturer's labeling, not studied

| Tolterodine (Detrol) | Immediate release: 1 and 2 mg; maximum, 4 mg daily
Extended release: 2 and 4 mg; maximum, 4 mg daily | >10%:
Gastrointestinal: xerostomia (35%; extended-release capsules: 23%)

1%–10%:
Cardiovascular: chest pain (2%)
Central nervous system: headache (7%; extended-release capsules: 6%), dizziness (5%; extended-release capsules: 2%), fatigue (4%; extended-release capsules: 2%), drowsiness (immediate and extended release: 3%), anxiety (extended-release capsules: 1%)
Dermatologic: xeroderma (1%)
Endocrine and metabolic: weight gain (1%)
Gastrointestinal: constipation (7%; extended-release capsules: 6%), abdominal pain (5%; extended-release capsules: 4%), diarrhea (4%), dyspepsia (4%; extended-release capsules: 3%)
Genitourinary: dysuria (2%; extended-release capsules: 1%)
Infection: infection (1%)
Neuromuscular and skeletal: arthralgia (2%)
Ophthalmic: xerophthalmia (immediate and extended release: 3%), visual disturbance (2%; extended-release capsules: 1%)
Respiratory: flulike symptoms (3%), bronchitis (2%), sinusitis (extended-release capsules: 2%) | Immediate-release tablet
CrCl 10–30 mL/min: 1 mg twice daily; use with caution
Extended-release capsule
CrCl 10–30 mL/min: 2 mg once daily
CrCl <10 mL/min: use is not recommended; has not been studied |

(continued on next page)

Table 5
(continued)

Medication	Dosage	Adverse Reactions	Renal Dosing
Darifenacin (Enablex)	7.5 and 15 mg extended-release tablet	>10%: Gastrointestinal: xerostomia (19%–35%), constipation (15%–21%) 1%–10%: Cardiovascular: hypertension (≥1%), peripheral edema (≥1%) Central nervous system: headache (7%), dizziness (<2%), pain (≥1%) Dermatologic: pruritus (≥1%), skin rash (≥1%), xeroderma (≥1%) Endocrine and metabolic: weight gain (≥1%) Gastrointestinal: dyspepsia (3%–8%), abdominal pain (2%–4%), nausea (2%–4%), vomiting (≥1%) Genitourinary: UTI (4%–5%), vaginitis (≥1%), urinary retention (acute) Neuromuscular and skeletal: weakness (<3%), arthralgia (≥1%), back pain (≥1%) Ophthalmic: dry eye syndrome (2%), visual disturbance (≥1%) Respiratory: flulike symptoms (1%–3%), bronchitis (≥1%), pharyngitis (≥1%), rhinitis (≥1%), sinusitis (≥1%)	No dosage adjustment necessary
Solifenacin (VESIcare)	5 and 10 mg	>10%: Gastrointestinal: xerostomia (11%–28%; dose related), constipation (5%–13%; dose related) 1%–10%: Cardiovascular: edema (≤1%), hypertension (≤1%) Central nervous system: fatigue (1%–2%), depression (≤1%) Gastrointestinal: dyspepsia (1%–4%), nausea (2%–3%), upper abdominal pain (1%–2%) Genitourinary: UTI (3%–5%), urinary retention (≤1%) Ophthalmic: blurred vision (4%–5%), dry eye syndrome (≤2%) Respiratory: cough (≤1%) Miscellaneous: influenza (≤2%)	CrCl ≥30 mL/min: there are no dosage adjustments provided in the manufacturer's labeling; use with caution CrCl <30 mL/min: maximum dose: 5 mg/d

| Fesoterodine (Toviaz) | 4 and 8 mg extended-release tablet | >10%:
  Gastrointestinal: xerostomia (19%–35%; dose related)
1%–10%:
  Cardiovascular: peripheral edema (1%)
  Central nervous system: insomnia (1%)
  Dermatologic: skin rash (1%)
  Endocrine and metabolic: increased gamma-glutamyl transferase level (1%)
  Gastrointestinal: constipation (4%–6%), dyspepsia (2%), nausea (1%–2%), abdominal pain (1%)
  Genitourinary: UTI (3%–4%), dysuria (1%–2%), urinary retention (1%)
  Hepatic: increased serum alanine transaminase level (1%)
  Neuromuscular and skeletal: back pain (1%–2%)
  Ophthalmic: dry eye syndrome (1%–4%)
  Respiratory: upper respiratory tract infection (2%–3%), cough (1%–2%), dry throat (1%–2%) | CrCl ≥30 mL/min: no dosage adjustment necessary
CrCl <30 mL/min: 4 mg once daily; maximum dose, 4 mg once daily |
| Trospium (Sanctura) | Immediate release: 20 mg twice daily
Extended release: 60 mg once daily in the morning | >10%:
  Gastrointestinal: xerostomia (9%–22%)
1%–10%:
  Cardiovascular: tachycardia (<2%)
  Central nervous system: headache (4%–7%), fatigue (2%)
  Dermatologic: skin rash (<2%), xeroderma
  Gastrointestinal: constipation (9%–10%), abdominal pain (1%–3%), dyspepsia (1%–2%), flatulence (1%–2%), abdominal distention (<2%), nausea (1%), dysgeusia, vomiting
  Genitourinary: UTI (1%–7%), urinary retention (≤1%)
  Infection: influenza (2%)
  Ophthalmic: dry eye syndrome (1%–2%), blurred vision (1%)
  Respiratory: nasopharyngitis (3%), dry nose (1%) | CrCl ≥30 mL/min: no dosage adjustment provided in manufacturer's labeling; renal impairment increases systemic exposure to trospium. Monitor for increased adverse effects
CrCl <30 mL/min:
  Immediate release: 20 mg once daily at bedtime
  Extended release: use not recommended |

Table 6
Miscellaneous

Medication	Dosage	Adverse Reactions	Renal Dosing
Tadalafil (Cialis)	2.5 and 5 mg	>10%: Cardiovascular: flushing (1%–13%; dose related) Central nervous system: headache (3%–42%; dose related), limb pain (1%–11%) Gastrointestinal: dyspepsia (1%–13%), nausea (10%–11%) Neuromuscular and skeletal: myalgia (1%–14%; dose related), back pain (2%–12%) Respiratory: respiratory tract infection (3%–13%), nasopharyngitis (2%–13%) 1%–10%: Cardiovascular: hypertension (1%–3%), angina pectoris (<2%), chest pain (<2%), facial edema (<2%), hypotension (<2%), myocardial infarction (<2%), orthostatic hypotension (<2%), palpitations (<2%), peripheral edema (<2%), syncope (<2%), tachycardia (<2%) Central nervous system: dizziness (<2%), drowsiness (<2%), fatigue (<2%), hypoesthesia (<2%), insomnia (<2%), pain (<2%), paresthesia (<2%), vertigo (<2%) Dermatologic: diaphoresis (<2%), pruritus (<2%), skin rash (<2%)	CrCl ≥51 mL/min: no dosage adjustment necessary CrCl 30–50 mL/min: initial, 2.5 mg once daily; maximum, 5 mg once daily CrCl <30 mL/min: use not recommended

Endocrine and metabolic: increased gamma-glutamyl transferase level (<2%)

Gastrointestinal: gastroenteritis (viral, 3%–5%), gastroesophageal reflux disease (1%–3%), abdominal pain (1%–2%), diarrhea (1%–2%), dysphagia (<2%), esophagitis (<2%), gastritis (<2%), hemorrhoidal bleeding (<2%), loose stools (<2%), upper abdominal pain (<2%), vomiting (<2%), xerostomia (<2%)

Genitourinary: spontaneous erections (<2%), UTI (≤2%)

Hematologic and oncologic: rectal hemorrhage (<2%)

Hepatic: abnormal liver function tests (<2%)

Neuromuscular and skeletal: arthralgia (<2%), neck pain (<2%), weakness (<2%)

Ophthalmic: blurred vision (<2%), conjunctival hyperemia (<2%), conjunctivitis (<2%), eye pain (<2%), lacrimation (<2%), periorbital swelling (<2%), vision color changes (<2%)

Otic: hearing loss (<2%), tinnitus (<2%)

Renal: renal insufficiency (<2%)

Respiratory: nasal congestion (≤9%), flulike symptoms (2%–5%), cough (2%–4%), bronchitis (≤2%), dyspnea (<2%), epistaxis (<2%), pharyngitis (<2%)

(continued on next page)

Table 6
(continued)

Medication	Dosage	Adverse Reactions	Renal Dosing

Mirabegron (Myrbetriq)	25 and 50 mg extended-release tablet	>10%:
		  Cardiovascular: hypertension (9%–11%)
		1%–10%:
		  Cardiovascular: tachycardia (2%)
		  Central nervous system: headache (4%), dizziness (3%)
		  Gastrointestinal: constipation (2%–3%), xerostomia (3%), diarrhea (2%), abdominal pain (1%)
		  Genitourinary: UTI (3%–6%), cystitis (2%)
		  Infection: influenza (3%)
		  Neuromuscular and skeletal: back pain (3%), arthralgia (2%)
		  Respiratory: nasopharyngitis (4%), sinusitis (3%)
			CrCl 30–89 mL/min or eGFR 30–89 mL/min/1.73 m²: no dosage adjustment necessary
			CrCl 15–29 mL/min or eGFR 15–29 mL/min/1.73 m²: do not exceed 25 mg once daily
			CrCl <15 mL/min or eGFR <15 mL/min/1.73 m²: not recommended (has not been studied)

Abbreviation: eGFR, estimated glomerular filtration rate.

- Holmium laser resection of the prostate
- Photoselective vaporization of the prostate
- Transurethral incision of the prostate
- Transurethral vaporization of the prostate
- Transurethral resection of the prostate (TURP)
  - Monopolar
  - Bipolar
- Open prostatectomy

AUA guidelines state that, "surgery is recommended for patients who have renal insufficiency secondary to BPH [benign prostatic hyperplasia], who have recurrent UTIs, bladder stones or gross hematuria due to BPH, and those who have LUTS refractory to other therapies."[5] Surgical planning depends on the clinical situation, the patient's anatomy, surgeon expertise, and equipment available. The discussion on pros/cons of each of the minimally invasive and surgical options is beyond the scope of this article. The 2003 AUA guidelines recognized TURP as the benchmark for therapy; however, emerging technologies for endoscopic management of the prostate give patients many options and discussion with a urologic specialist helps to tailor the menu of choices to the best option for the individual patient.

SUMMARY

Effective evaluation, treatment, and management of male LUTS should be initiated in the primary care setting using the tools outlined not only in this article but in this issue as a whole. A thorough history and physical examination with limited laboratory testing and special testing easily guides PAs to prescribe medical therapy and advise the patient how long it may take to achieve a response. It is important to evaluate for comorbid ED in this disease state and can assist in medication choices and serve as motivation for treating LUTS and ED. Specialty referral should be reserved for patients who are refractory to medical management, desire surgical management, have an initial abnormal laboratory evaluation (PSA and UA) or physical examination, those in urinary retention, and those with high index of suspicion for urethral stricture disease. Using the strategies discussed here should lessen the anxiety associated with evaluating men with urinary symptoms and provide the ability to initiate medical therapy in a logical stepwise manner.

REFERENCES

1. Abrams P, Chapple C, Khoury S, et al. Evaluation and treatment of lower urinary tract symptoms in older men. J Urol 2009;181:1779.
2. Kirby M, Chapple C, Jackson G, et al. Erectile dysfunction and lower urinary tract symptoms: a consensus on the importance of co-diagnosis. Int J Clin Pract 2013; 67(7):606–18.
3. Seftel AD, De la Rosette J, Birt J, et al. Coexisting lower urinary tract symptoms and erectile dysfunction: a systematic review of epidemiological data. Int J Clin Pract 2013;67(1):32–45.
4. Barry MJ, Fowler FJ, O'Leary MP, et al, Measurement Committee of the American Urological Association. The American Urological Association symptom index for benign prostatic hyperplasia. J Urol 2017;197(2):S189–97.
5. McVary KT, Roehrborn CG, & Avins AL. Management of benign prostatic hyperplasia (BPH). American Urological Association website. 2010. Available at: http://

www.auanet.org/content/guidelines-and-quality-care/clinical-guidelines.cfm. Accessed August 25, 2017.

6. Rosen RC, Riley A, Wagner G, et al. The International Index of Erectile Function (IIEF): a multidimensional scale for assessment of erectile dysfunction. Urology 1997;49(6):822–30.

7. McConnell JD, Roehrborn CG, Bautista OM, et al, Medical Therapy of Prostatic Symptoms (MTOPS) Research Group. The long-term effect of doxazosin, finasteride, and combination therapy on the clinical progression of benign prostatic hyperplasia. N Engl J Med 2003;349(25):2387–98.

8. Siami P, Roehrborn CG, Barkin J, et al, CombAT study group. Combination therapy with dutasteride and tamsulosin in men with moderate-to-severe benign prostatic hyperplasia and prostate enlargement: the CombAT (Combination of Avodart® and Tamsulosin) trial rationale and study design. Contemp Clin Trials 2007;28(6):770–9.

9. Porru D, Jallous H, Cavalli V, et al. Prognostic value of a combination of IPSS, flow rate and residual urine volume compared to pressure-flow studies in the preoperative evaluation of symptomatic BPH. Eur Urol 2002;41(3):246–9.

10. American Geriatrics Society 2015 Beers Criteria Update Expert Panel. American Geriatrics Society 2015 Updated Beers Criteria for potentially inappropriate medication use in older adults. J Am Geriatr Soc 2015;63:2227–46.

11. Barry MJ. Epidemiology and natural history of benign prostatic hyperplasia. Urol Clin North Am 1990;17:495.

12. Barry MJ. Medical outcomes research and benign prostatic hyperplasia. Prostate 1990;3(suppl):61.

13. Lepor H. Nonoperative management of benign prostatic hyperplasia. J Urol 1989; 141:1283.

14. Lexi-Comp. Drug Information Handbook: A Clinically Relevant Resource for All Healthcare Professionals. 26th edition. Hudson (OH): Wolters Kluwer; 2017.

Neurogenic Bladder and Its Management

Jessica Nelson, MPAS, PA-C

KEYWORDS

- Neurogenic bladder • Voiding dysfunction • Cerebrovascular accident
- Parkinson disease • Cerebral palsy • Spinal cord injury • Multiple sclerosis
- Transverse myelitis

KEY POINTS

- Neurogenic bladder dysfunction can be caused by several neurologic conditions.
- It is important to recognize patients with neuropathic voiding dysfunction to manage any upper tract damage that can occur as a result.
- Treatment of neuropathic voiding dysfunction is aimed at maintaining adequate storage and drainage in a low-pressure system without upper tract damage or infection while maintaining continence
- Goals of therapy also include improving patient quality of life.

BACKGROUND

The functions of the lower urinary tract (LUT) are to store and eliminate urine. This is a coordinated behavior between the brain, spinal cord, urinary bladder, and outlet. For the bladder to empty, the bladder contracts, which is under control of the parasympathetic system, in coordination with relaxation of the sphincter, under control of the somatic nervous system. Disturbances in the nervous system that controls the LUT can lead to neuropathic voiding dysfunction or neurogenic bladder (NGB). NGB is a term used to denote LUT symptoms (LUTS) as a sequela of neurologic disease. It is important to recognize patients at risk because long-term effects of NGB can result in later upper tract dysfunction and renal damage and concomitant LUT deterioration. The risk of developing upper tract damage is highest in patients with traumatic neurologic disorders, such as spinal cord injury (SCI) and spina bifida, versus nontraumatic slow progressive disorders.[1] Other complications of having an NGB include hydronephrosis, urinary tract infections, and urinary calculi. Thus, it is important to keep in mind that these patients can also experience sexual dysfunction.

Disclosure Statement: The authors have nothing to disclose.
Department of Urology, UT Southwestern Medical Center, 5323 Harry Hines Boulevard, Dallas, TX 75390, USA
E-mail address: Jessica.nelson@utsouthwestern.edu

Physician Assist Clin 3 (2018) 103–111
http://dx.doi.org/10.1016/j.cpha.2017.08.008
2405-7991/18/© 2017 Elsevier Inc. All rights reserved.

RISK FACTORS AND EPIDEMIOLOGY

Neuropathic voiding dysfunction can be caused by various diseases or events that affect the nervous systems controlling the LUT. The location of the extent of the neurologic lesion dictate the extent of LUT damage (European Association of Urology guidelines, 2017). NGB dysfunction may arise as a result of several neurologic conditions. NGB has been found in 40% to 90% of patients in the United States with multiple sclerosis (MS), 37% to 72% of patients with parkinsonism, and 15% of patients with stroke.[2,3] It is estimated that up to 70% to 84% of patients with SCI have some component of voiding dysfunction.[2,4] In a recent retrospective study performed by Bulent,[5] the median patient age for SCI was 33 years (ages ranged from 18–75). The leading causes of SCI were motor vehicle accidents (40%) and falls (29%). Upper urinary tract deterioration as a serious complication of NGB was determined in 25% of patients. Less common scenarios for NGB may include diabetes mellitus with autonomic neuropathy, complications from pelvic surgery, and cauda equine syndrome due to lumbar spine pathology.[2]

EXAMINATION

Patients with NGB can experience irritative voiding symptoms, such as urinary frequency, urgency, nocturia, and urgency incontinence. Early diagnosis and treatment are essential for prevention of all these conditions, requiring a detailed history and physical examination. These should include past and present symptoms. Attention to fluid intake, voiding habits, and presence of incontinence is important. Inclusion of a bowel history, obstetric history, and sexual history is also important because all histories can be affected. During examination, it is vital to examine a patient's back, looking for a sacral dimple or hair tuft that could be a sign of occult spina bifida. It is also important to perform a thorough neurologic examination to identify sensory or motor function deficits. If incomplete bladder emptying is suspected, then a post-void residual should be obtained because some patients may have incomplete voiding without appropriate sensation.

Laboratory Examination

Obtaining a urinalysis and urine culture is warranted; however, treatment of bacteriuria in patients with indwelling catheters or those performing intermittent self-catheterization is not routinely recommended for identification of asymptomatic bacteriuria given frequent colonization. Treatment in these patients is only recommended in the context of symptoms. Symptoms of UTI in these patients include fever, suprapubic pain, flank pain hematuria, abrupt change in continence, and autonomic dysreflexia (AD) in those susceptible. Urine odor is often an associated complaint; however, it must be accompanied by other symptoms, listed previously, and not treated in isolation. Other laboratory tests to be considered include serum creatinine and glomerular filtration rate to monitor renal function and prostate-specific antigen in appropriate patients.

Urodynamics

Urodynamics (UDS) provides a way to help evaluate and manage the bladder in patients with certain neurologic conditions. In a report by Kaplan and colleagues,[6] there was a general correlation between the neurologic level of injury and the expected vesicourethral function, but it was neither absolute nor specific, and UDS provides a more precise diagnosis for each patient. If there is any suspicion for upper tract deterioration from bladder symptomatology, then UDS is warranted.

DISEASES THAT CONTRIBUTE TO NEUROPATHIC VOIDING DYSFUNCTION
Cortical Lesions

The 3 diseases highlighted in this section are stroke, Parkinson disease, and cerebral palsy (CP). Patients with these lesions typically manifest involuntary bladder contractions with coordinated external sphincter and bladder neck activity. Sensation and voluntary striated sphincter function are typically preserved, but sensation may be deficient or delayed. Urinary incontinence may also be reported.[7]

Cerebrovascular Accident is a common deadly or debilitating event that can affect the brain. After the acute event, detrusor areflexia leads to urinary retention. It may take weeks to months for recovery to occur if this happens.[7] The initial work-up in these patients is a urinalysis and postvoid residual. Generally, sensation is still intact and patients may have urinary frequency and urgency secondary to detrusor overactivity (DO). If clinically warranted, cystoscopy and/or UDS can be used to further clarify treatment options, especially in elderly patients with other comorbidities that could contribute to other pathologies, such as bladder cancer or an enlarged prostate (see AUA core curriculum). For example, poor emptying in a man with LUTS prior to the event of stroke suggests prostatic obstruction as the primary cause. In select cases, it is advisable to rule out overactivity with impaired contractility with UDS to prevent a patient from undergoing a surgical outlet procedure that might not be beneficial.

Parkinson Disease

Parkinson disease is a neurodegenerative disorder that leads to progressive deterioration of motor function due to loss of dopamine neurons in the substantia nigra. Hallmark features of dopamine deficiency include skeletal rigidity, resting tremor, and bradykinesia. Patients with Parkinson disease often have LUTS. Most studies find an average of 5 years from the onset of PD to the initiation of LUTS. The most frequent symptoms include nocturia (86%), followed by urinary frequency (71%) and urgency (68%).[7] The most common urodynamic finding in patients with PD is DO. Urinary incontinence is found in approximately 1 in 4 patients, with 26% in symptomatic men and 28% of women with Parkinson disease.[8,9] Evaluation starting with urinalysis and postvoid residual is recommended whereas UDS is reserved for patients who fail medical therapy or in whom surgery might be considered. Although historically, patients with PD were discouraged from having a transurethral resection of the prostate due to sphincter concerns, those with clear bladder outlet obstruction on UDS can now be considered surgical candidates. Unlike some of the other disease conditions, patients with PD are at low risk of upper tract deterioration.

Cerebral Palsy

CP is a disorder of movement, posture, and muscle tone caused by damage to the immature brain, most often before birth. Due to varying severity and definition of the disease, the incidence of LUT dysfunction in the CP population is unknown. In a recent review of the literature by Samijn and colleagues,[10] however, it was found that 55% of patients with CP have LUTS with storage symptoms being the most common due to the high prevalence of neurogenic DO. Those with voiding symptoms and pelvic floor dysfunction are more prone to progress to upper urinary tract dysfunction later in life. In these patients UDS can help direct management. Further research on this topic is needed.

Disease Primarily Involving the Spinal Cord

Spinal cord injuries (SCIs), transverse myelitis (TM), spina bifida, and MS fall into this category. Bladder dysfunction in these patients depends on where the lesion is located. Complete lesions between level T6 and S2 usually exhibit absent sensation, involuntary bladder contractions, and smooth sphincter synergy, with striated sphincter dyssynergia. Patients with lesions above T6 may exhibit smooth sphincter dyssynergia and autonomic hyperreflexia. Urinary incontinence may also occur.[7]

A potentially serious clinical condition that can occur in patients with lesions above T6 is AD. AD is caused by unregulated sympathetic nervous system stimulation and is triggered by noxious afferent stimulation below the level of the injury. The most common urologic causes include urinary retention, urinary tract infection, and DO in the setting of low bladder compliance. It manifests as rapidly escalating hypertension (40 mm Hg above resting blood pressure), diaphoresis, and bradycardia.[11]

In an article by Milligan and colleagues,[12] a step-by-step approach is offered to aid during this situation:

1. Monitor patient heart rate and blood pressure every 5 minutes.
2. Remove tight clothing and straps.
3. Examine the bladder—if in urinary retention, immediately drain bladder via urethral catheter or by unplugging obstructed indwelling catheter.
4. Assess for constipation and fecal impaction.
5. If blood pressure continues to rise, the following medications may be administered:
   a. Nitroglycerine (0.4 mg sublingual every 5 minutes or 3.5-inches nitropaste to chest wall)
   b. Captopril 25 mg sublingual

SCI patients are at risk of impaired compliance, and detrusor sphincter dyssynergia (DSD) urodynamic evaluation is warranted.[13] Upper tract imaging for hydronephrosis or stone disease is also suggested as well as monitoring of renal function.

Spinal cord injuries

SCIs are most common in men, making up 80% of the injuries. (AUA Update on Urologic Management of Spinal Cord Injuries in 2008). In patients with a suprasacral SCI, there is an initial period of spinal shock that can occur, characterized by an acontractile bladder, absent sensation and closed proximal urethra and sphincter. The patient is continent but in urinary retention. This can last weeks to months, generally noted to be approximately 6 to 8 weeks, and during this time frame, UDS is not recommended.[14] Once there is recovery from spinal shock, there is spontaneous voiding or more commonly incontinence.[15] Although presentation is variable depending on the level and completeness of injury, many patients with suprasacral injuries (typically above T10) have DO on urodynamic studies. In general, most are also at risk for DSD, which is defined as intermittent or complete failure of relaxation of the urinary sphincter during a bladder contraction and voiding, resulting in sustained elevation in intravesical pressures and incomplete bladder emptying. Finally, low thoracic or sacral lesions can cause an acontractile bladder with an intact external sphincter. Patients with incomplete injuries may have a variety of findings, including altered compliance, which can result in upper tract deterioration with time, even in the absence of notable symptoms.[15,16]

Multiple sclerosis

MS is an autoimmune demyelinating disease of the central nervous system that affects how the brain communicates with the body. This can lead to bladder dysfunction in several ways. MS has a median global incidence of 2.5 per 100,000 (range 1.1–4).[17] Median prevalence is in the United States is 135 per 100,000. Most commonly the age of onset is 30 years to 38 years of age for relapsing, remitting, and progressive phases. Common symptoms of the disease include optic nerve dysfunction, pyramidal tract abnormalities (hyperreflexia), ataxia, bowel dysfunction, NGB, and bowel and sexual dysfunction. Primary and secondary progressive MS are predominantly spinal diseases, and their activity affects LUT function.[7] More than 80% of patients with MS report genitourinary symptoms, with voiding dysfunction having an impact on the vast majority of these patients.[18,19] A variety of voiding complaints are seen, with DO of the bladder noted in 50% to 90% of patients with MS and detrusor areflexia in 20% to 30% of patients with MS.[2,3] Neurogenic DO is the most common urodynamic finding found in patients with MS.[20] This is seen in up to 99% of patients, and DSD and detrusor hypocontractility are seen in up to 83% and 40% of these patients, respectively.[21]

In contrast to patients with traumatic SCI, MS patients with neurogenic voiding dysfunction seem to be at a low risk for upper urinary tract deterioration.[1] Those at higher risk for upper tract abnormality, however, include men and those with altered compliance; therefore, they should undergo periodic upper tract imaging and likely closer after with urodynamic testing.[22]

Transverse myelitis

TM is a heterogenous syndrome characterized by acute or subacute spinal cord dysfunction resulting in paresis, sensory deficit, and frequently autonomic (bladder, bowel, and sexual) impairment.[23] The annual incidence of TM is estimated to be 1.34 to 4.60 cases per million people. The exact etiology is unknown. The initial presentation can occur at any age, and urinary symptoms most often present as retention during the acute stage.[23,24] Multiple studies have shown that even after spinal cord inflammation resolves and neurologic recovery occurs, patients may continue to have bladder and sexual symptoms.[23–29] Over time, patients often also develop urinary urgency often with incontinence.

Many series have demonstrated patients with TM to have DO, DSD, and detrusor underactivity on UDS, although series are generally small with short follow-up.[23,30] Decreased compliance and upper tract damage have also been noted in this patient population.[29] Due to the risk of upper tract damage, patients should undergo not only urodynamic testing but also upper tract imaging with renal sonogram.[31]

Spina bifida

Spina bifida occurs when there is incomplete neural closure during the first trimester of pregnancy. The birth prevalence of spina bifida in the United States is currently approximately 30 per 100,000. Generally, voiding dysfunction begins at an early age but can be delayed until adulthood. Video-urodynamic studies can identify a variety of features, such as DO, detrusor underactivity, or low compliance with ineffective contractions.

Monitoring of patients from infancy is recognized as important for long-term renal preservation and continence. Controversy continues, however, regarding the optimal use and timing of urodynamic studies and the indications for initiation of clean intermittent catheterization and anticholinergics in infants and children.[32] Closer monitoring in recent years has brought timely interventions that have increased patients' lifespan. In addition, in utero intervention may improve patient outcomes, although conflicting data exist.[33] Treatment of patients with spina bifida is based on results of UDS, renal function, continence, and the presence of recurrent UTIs.

DISEASE DISTAL TO THE SPINAL CORD

Diabetes mellitus as well as cauda equine syndrome and sequela of pelvic surgery fall under this category. Patients with any of these diseases may be areflexic or underactive detrusor with denervated/underactive external sphincter but coordinated bladder neck (neurology of bladder, bowel, and sexual dysfunction). Also notable is that these patients can have sensory impairment as well as incontinence. The classic symptoms of diabetic bladder dysfunction include decreased bladder sensation, increased bladder capacity, and impaired bladder emptying with resultant elevated postvoid residual urine.

TREATMENT OF VOIDING DYSFUNCTION AND GOALS OF MANAGEMENT

The goals of treatment of patients with an NGB are to maintain adequate storage and drainage in a low pressure system without upper tract damage or infection while maintaining continence (**Box 1**). When managing any of these patients, it is vital to take into account disease progression, comorbidities, manual dexterity, mobility, and family and social support systems.

Behavioral measures are most valuable in patients who have some degree of bladder control and intact bladder sensation. This has been found helpful for patients with neurologic lesions involving the brain, such as cerebrovascular disease, Parkinson disease, multiple system atrophy, dementia, and CP as well as for patients with MS, incomplete SCI, TM, and diabetes mellitus.[34,35]

The mainstay of options for patients with NGB includes anticholinergics with or without use of clean intermittent catheterization. Although anticholinergics are recommended as first-line pharmacologic treatment of urinary symptoms, many patients have an inadequate response and/or experience intolerable adverse effects.[36] Combination therapy using 2 or 3 different oral agents (antimuscarinics, α-blockers, and tricyclic antidepressants) has been found effective in patients with NGB and poor bladder compliance.[37] Although not approved for this use, β_3-adrenergic agonists (mirabegron) could also be helpful for neurogenic DO. It is currently approved and vastly studied in overactive bladder. Specifically, in patients with Parkinson disease, mirabegron may be a good alternative due to anticholinergic side effects commonly seen as a result of concurrent antiparkinson medications.

Second-line treatments for NGB include neuromodulation (sacral neuromodulation), botulinum toxin A (Botox) injection, indwelling catheters (urethral or suprapubic), and in select cases surgery. Sacral nerve modulation has been used to treat overactive bladder and has been approved by the Food and Drug Administration for treatment of urge incontinence, urinary urgency and frequency, and nonobstructive urinary retention. Sacral neuromodulation has not been approved by the FDA for NGB, although it has been investigated for the treatment of it. The mechanism of action for onabotulinum toxin A (Botox) includes reducing bladder contractility by inhibiting presynaptic release of acetylcholine from nerve terminals through binding of SNAP-

---

Box 1
Goals of management

Preserve renal function

Absence or control of infection

Adequate storage at low intravesical pressure

Adequate emptying at low intravesical pressure

Achieve and maintain continence

Optimize quality of life

25, thus reducing stimulation of the muscarinic receptors.[38] Data from a double-blind, randomized trial of MS and SCI NGB patients suggested the number of incontinence episodes significantly decreased (an average of 21 for 200 units and 23 for 300 units) 6 weeks after onabotulinum toxin A injections.[39]

When chronic catheterization is required, suprapubic management is preferable to indwelling urethral catheterization. Clean intermittent self-catheterization, however, remains the gold standard.[40] In a retrospective study of 308 SCI patients followed over 18 years, upper tract changes were more frequent in patients with indwelling catheters (18%) compared with those using intermittent catheterization (6.5%).[41]

REFERENCES

1. Lawrenson R, Wyndaele JJ, Vlachonikolis I, et al. Renal failure in patients with neurogenic lower urinary tract dysfunction. Neuroepidemiology 2001;20:138–43.
2. Dorsher PT, McIntosh PM. Neurogenic bladder. Adv Urol 2012;2012:816274.
3. Lansang RS, Krouskop AC. Bladder management. In: Massagli TL, et al, editors. eMedicine; 2004.
4. Manack A, Mostko SP, Haag-Molkenteller C, et al. Epidemiology and healthcare utilization of neurogenic bladder patients in a US claims database. Neurourol Urodyn 2011;30:395–401.
5. Bulent C. Risk factors predicting upper urinary tract deterioration in patients with spinal cord injury: a retrospective study. Neurourol Urodyn 2017;36:653–8.
6. Kaplan SA, Chancellor MB, Blaivas JG. Bladder and sphincter behavior in patients with spinal cord lesions. J Urol 1991;146:113–7.
7. Wein A, Kavoussi L, Partin A, Campbell Walsh Urology, 11th edition. Philadelphia: Elsevier; 2015. p. 1761-95.
8. Sakakibara R, Tateno F, Nagao T, et al. Bladder function of patients with Parkinson's disease. Int J Urol 2014;21:638–46.
9. Sakakibara R, Panicker J, Finazzi-Agro E, et al. A guideline for the management of bladder dysfunction in Parkinson's disease and other gait disorders. Neurourol Urodyn 2016;35(5):551–63.
10. Samijn B, Van Laecke E, Renson C, et al. Lower urinary tract symptoms and urodynamic findings in children and adults with cerebral palsy: A systematic review. Neurourol Urodyn 2017;36(3):541–9.
11. Trop CS, Bennett CJ. Autonomic dysreflexia and its urological implications: a review. J Urol 1991;146:1461–9.
12. Milligan J, Lee J, McMillan C, et al. Autonomic dysreflexia: recognizing a common serious condition in patients with spinal cord injury. Can Fam Physician 2012; 58(8):831–5.
13. Schops TF, Schneider MP, Steffen F, et al. Neurogenic lower urinary tract dysfunction in patient with spinal cord injury long-term urodynamics findings. BJU Int 2015;115(suppl 6):33–8.
14. Chancellor MR. Urodynamic evaluation after spinal cord injury. Phys Med Rehabil Clin N Am 1993;4:273–98.
15. Harris C, Lemack G. Neurourologic dysfunction: evaluation, surveillance and therapy. Current Opinion in Urology 2016;26(4):290–4.
16. Consortium for Spinal Cord Medicine. Bladder management for adults with spinal cord injury: a clinical practice guideline for health-care providers. J Spinal Cord Med 2006;29:527–73.

17. World Health Organization. Atlas: multiple sclerosis resources in the world. 2008. Available at: http://www.who.int/mental_health/neurology/Atlas_MS_WEB.pdf. Accessed June 21, 2017.

18. Pentyala S, Jalali S, Park J, et al. Urologic problems in multiple sclerosis. Open Androl J 2010;2:37–41.

19. Litwiller SE, Frohman ER, Zimmern PE. Multiple sclerosis andthe urologist. J Urol 1999;161:743–57.

20. Dillon BE, Lemack GE. Urodynamics in the evaluation of the patient with multiple sclerosis: when are they helpful and how do we use them? Urol Clin North Am 2014;41(3):439–44.

21. De Seze M, Ruffion A, Denys P, et al. The neurogenic bladder in multiple sclerosis: review of the literature and proposal of management guidelines. Mult Scler 2007;13:915–28.

22. Groen J, Pannek J, Castro Diaz D, et al. Summary of European association of urology (EAU) guidelines on neuro-urology. Eur Urol 2016;69:324–33.

23. Beh SC, Greenberg BM, Frohman T, et al. Transverse myelitis. Neurol Clin 2013; 31:79–138.

24. Kalita J, Shah S, Kapoor R, et al. Bladder dysfunction in acute transverse myelitis: magnetic resonance imaging and neurophysiological and urodynamic correlations. J Neurol Neurosurg Psychiatry 2002;73:154–9.

25. Berger Y, Blaivas JG, Oliver L. Urinary dysfunction in transverse myelitis. J Urol 1990;144:103–5.

26. Cheng W, Chiu R, Tam P. Residual bladder dysfunction 2 to 10 years after acute transverse myelitis. J Paediatr Child Health 1999;35:476–8.

27. Ganesan V, Borzyskowski M. Characteristics and course of urinary tract dysfunction after acute transverse myelitis in. Dev Med Child Neurol 2001;43:473–5.

28. Sakakibara R, Hattori T, Yasuda K, et al. Micturition disturbance in acute transverse myelitis. Spinal Cord 1996;34:481–5.

29. Tanaka ST, Stone AR, Kurzrock EA. Transverse myelitis in children: long-term urological outcomes. J Urol 2006;175:1865–8 [discussion:8].

30. Frohman EM, Wingerchuk DM. Clinical practice. Transverse myelitis. N Engl J Med 2010;363:564–72.

31. Gliga LA, Lavelle RS, Christie AL, et al. Urodynamics findings in transverse myelitis patients with lower urinary tract symptoms: results from a tertiary referral urodynamic center. Neurourol Urodyn 2017;36:360–3.

32. Snow-Lisy DC, Yerkes EB, Cheng EY. Update on urological management of spina bifida from prenatal diagnosis to adulthood. J Urol 2015;194:288–96.

33. Brock JW 3rd, Carr MC, Adzick NS, et al. Bladder function after fetal surgery for myelomeningocele. Pediatrics 2015;136:e906–13. Important follow up of the MOMS trial showing no clear urologic benefit to antenatal myelomeningocele closure.

34. Wyndaele J-J. Conservative treatment of patients with neurogenicbladder. Eur Urol Suppl 2008;7:557–65.

35. Hadley EC. Bladder training and related therapies for urinary incontinence in older people. JAMA 1986;256:372–9.

36. Chapple CR, Khullar V, Gabriel Z, et al. The effects of antimuscarinic treatments in overactive bladder: an update of a systematic review and meta-analysis. Eur Urol 2008;54:543–62.

37. Cameron AP, Clemens JQ, Latini JM, et al. Combination therapy improves compliance of the neurogenic bladder. J Urol 2009;182:1062–7.

38. Cruz F. Targets for botulinum toxin in the lower urinary tract. Neurourol Urodyn 2014;33(1):31–8.
39. Ginsberg D, Gousse A, Keppenne V, et al. Phase 3 efficacy and tolerability study of onabotulinumtoxinA for urinary incontinence from neurogenic detrusor overactivity. J Urol 2012;187(6):2131–9.
40. Stöhrer M, Blok B, Castro-Diaz D, et al. EAU guidelines on neurogenic lower urinary tract dysfunction. Eur Urol 2009;56:81–8. Available at: https://doi.org/10.1016/j.eururo.2009.04.028. Accessed July 26, 2017.
41. Cameron AP, Wallner LP, Tate DG, et al. Bladder management after spinal cord injury in the United States 1972 to 2005. J Urol 2010;184(1):213–7.

Erectile Dysfunction

Patrick Dougherty, MPAS, PA-C

KEYWORDS

- Erectile dysfunction • Impotence • Sexual dysfunction • PDE-5 inhibitors

KEY POINTS

- Erectile dysfunction (ED), although recognized as a pathologic condition for thousands of years, was not clearly defined until 1992, thus overcoming one of many barriers to treatment.
- ED is defined as the inability to achieve and/or maintain erection of sufficient rigidity and duration to permit satisfactory sexual performance.
- Causes of ED are psychogenic, vasculogenic, neurogenic, endocrinologic, cavernosal smooth muscle dysfunction, iatrogenic, or pharmacologic; for many patients the cause may be any combination of these.
- Diagnosis and evaluation of ED can be as simple as using a questionnaire but can also involve complex testing and imaging modalities, with varying degrees of reliability and clinical utility.
- Treatment of ED usually follows a stepwise progression, from noninvasive strategies, such as lifestyle modifications and oral medications, all the way to surgical placement of penile prostheses for severe refractory disease.

HISTORY

Although recognized as a pathologic condition for several millennia, the systematic and evidence-based investigation of erectile dysfunction (ED) is a relatively recent phenomenon in modern medicine. For as long as humans have been studying their sexuality, they have also been documenting the affliction of sexual dysfunction. By 1150 BCE, the ancient Egyptians had described 12 different sexual positions with explicit papyrus drawings that were passed down, studied, annotated, and preserved throughout the centuries. Predating these drawings by several hundred years, the Ebers papyrus contains, among many other remedies, prescriptions for "weakness of the male member" (1700 BCE).[1] Yet it was not until 1992 that the National Institutes of Health held a multidisciplinary consensus conference on impotence and officially defined ED as the inability to achieve and/or maintain erection of sufficient rigidity and duration to permit satisfactory sexual performance.[2] This marked a turning point

Department of Urology, UT Southwestern Medical Center, 5323 Harry Hines Boulevard, Dallas, TX 75390-9110, USA
E-mail address: Patrick.dougherty@utsouthwestern.edu

Physician Assist Clin 3 (2018) 113–127
http://dx.doi.org/10.1016/j.cpha.2017.08.011
2405-7991/18/© 2017 Elsevier Inc. All rights reserved.

for physicians and patients, making it easier to identify, diagnose, and address ED in common medical practice.

EPIDEMIOLOGY AND RISK FACTORS

The Massachusetts Male Aging Study (MMAS) was the first cross-sectional population study for prevalence of ED, taking a random sample of men in Boston, ages 40 to 70, and using a self-administered sexual activity questionnaire to stratify mild, moderate, and complete ED. Overall prevalence of ED, regardless of type and severity, was 52% in this cohort, and prevalence of complete ED increased from 5.1% in men age 40% to 15% in the 70-year-old group. The probability of moderate ED increased from 17% to 34% with age, and the prevalence of mild ED stayed at 17% regardless of age.[3] More recent data from the Boston Area Community Health Survey, 2005 to 2006, revealed 10% of men in their 30s compared with 59% of men in their 70s had ED.[4] Worldwide prevalence of ED was estimated at 5% to 28% based on the Global Survey of Sexual Attitudes and Behaviors, which included men and women ages 40 to 80 from 29 different countries.[5] The MMAS data from 1987 to 1989 was later compared with new data collected from 1995 to 1997, representing the first reported longitudinal data set for establishing incidence of ED. The study concluded risk of ED was approximately 26 new cases per 1000 men annually. There was a higher incidence in older men (46.4/1000 in men 60–69) and in men with cardiovascular disease (58.3/1000), hypertension (42.5/1000), and diabetes (50.7/1000). Other independent risk factors for ED include smoking, obesity, depressive symptoms, metabolic syndrome, hyperlipidemia, sedentary lifestyle, spinal cord injury, certain medications, neurodegenerative diseases, renal insufficiency, prostate cancer treatments, blunt perineal or pelvic trauma, and bicycle riding.[6–12]

ERECTILE PHYSIOLOGY

Normally, blood supply to the penis arises from the internal pudendal artery, which branches from the internal iliac artery, although there is often collateral circulation with accessory pudendal branches arising from other pelvic arteries, such as the external iliac, obturator, vesical, and femoral arteries.[13] The internal pudendal artery eventually becomes the common penile artery, which then branches into dorsal, bulbourethral, and cavernous arteries. The dorsal artery supplies the glans, and the cavernous artery is responsible for erection as it supplies the corpora cavernosa filling all of the branching helicine arteries, trabecular erectile tissue, and the sinusoids housed as a matrix of elastic erectile tissue within the cylindrical bilayered tunica albuginea. The outer layer of the tunica consists of collagen and elastin fibers arranged in a longitudinal fashion and the inner layer of circular-running fibers. On the periphery of the cavernosal sinusoids, there are subtunical venous plexuses, which drain venous blood and give rise to the emissary veins that penetrate through the tunical layers out to the larger return vessels.[14]

At baseline, the trabecular smooth muscle matrix of the corpus cavernosum is in a state of moderate tonic contraction, thus limiting arterial inflow and maintaining flaccidity. When the smooth muscle is further contracted, as in cold temperatures, the blood flow is further limited, resulting in shrinkage of the phallus. During erection, sexual stimulation via both somatic and autonomic pathways causes release of several neurotransmitters, including dopamine, serotonin, oxytocin, and, most importantly, nitric oxide (NO).[15] NO is responsible for binding and activating guanylyl cyclase, the enzyme that catalyzes the transition of guanosine 5′-triphosphate (GTP) to cyclic guanine monophosphate (cGMP), which relaxes cavernous smooth muscle.

NO released by neurons is responsible for initiation of erection through this mechanism; however, maintenance of the erection is mediated primarily by NO synthesized by the vascular endothelial cells.[16] With smooth muscle relaxation, the trabecular erectile tissue and sinusoids fill with blood causing increased rigidity.[17] Compression of the subtunical venous plexuses limits outflow, and the emissary veins traversing through the tunical layers are essentially pinched off as the hemodynamic pressure increases, further inhibiting detumescence.[14]

Erection is maintained until cGMP is degraded by phosphodiesterase enzyme (PDE) and the smooth muscle regains its tone. Inhibiting PDE has, therefore, become a major target for pharmacologic therapy for ED.

ETIOLOGIES AND ASSOCIATED CONDITIONS

The causes of ED can be broadly categorized as either organic, psychogenic, or mixed. Etiologies of organic ED are subdivided into vasculogenic, neurogenic, endocrinologic, and cavernosal smooth muscle dysfunction. Additionally, ED is also a result of iatrogenic trauma and medications.

Psychogenic ED stems from the release of adrenaline associated with psychologic stress. Many psychologic conditions have been implicated in ED, including depression, generalized anxiety, guilt, performance anxiety, relationship discord, and internal conflict about sexuality.[18] Sympathetic stress response stimulates catecholamine release, resulting in a shunting of blood flow away from the genitals and out to skeletal muscles in preparation for a fight-or-flight response, thus inhibiting penile tumescence. This adrenaline-mediated mechanism is particularly useful in explaining to patients why the excitement and anxiety experienced with a new sexual partner may result in premature loss of erection. It is also likely responsible for compounding the severity of ED in men with only mild vasculogenic or neurogenic pathology or in men who have lost an erection even 1 time who then experience sudden and severe ED in subsequent attempts despite no acute change in any other risk factors.[19]

Vasculogenic ED has been widely recognized as an early warning sign for underlying subclinical cardiovascular disease because both processes typically result from endothelial injury and dysfunction, which then progress to arterial insufficiency and vascular occlusive disease. Therefore, the independent risk factors commonly listed for coronary artery disease (CAD) are the same as for ED: blood pressure greater than 130/85, triglycerides greater than 150 mg/dL, high-density lipoprotein less than 40 mg/dL, diabetes, body mass index (BMI) over 30, waist circumference greater than 40 inches, tobacco use, and sedentary lifestyle.[6–12] Another important factor in vasculogenic ED is the reduced availability of endothelial NO seen with aging and in certain disease states, such as diabetes and sickle cell disease. This mechanism is the focus of many new and ongoing studies.[20–23]

Neurogenic ED is a broad category encompassing any insult to the nervous system, resulting in ED from chronic neurodegenerative conditions, such as Alzheimer disease, multiple sclerosis, acute injuries from spinal cord trauma, and stroke. Strokes involving the right occipitoparietal and thalamic areas may interfere with visual and somatosensory processing; and lesions involving the left insular and adjacent parietotemporal areas may disrupt the ability to generate visceral arousal states. These types of strokes have been shown to significantly reduce erectile function independent of age, stroke severity, infarct volume, brain volume, and independent CAD risk factors.[24] Spinal injury affecting the S2-4 nerve roots or downstream injury to the cavernous nerve often lead to ED. These injuries may be insidious from diabetic neuropathy or aging but often are acute injuries as a result of pelvic surgery, most commonly radical prostatectomy, although this is far less common with newer nerve-sparing techniques. Diabetes also commonly affects autonomic nerve function by progressive demyelination of peripheral nerves, including the cavernosal nerve. Denervation of the corpora cavernosa induces remodeling of the cavernosal sinusoids and smooth muscle complex, resulting in irreversible fibrosis and loss of compliance and elasticity needed for penile tumescence and rigidity.

Endocrinologic ED primarily refers to hypogonadism or testosterone deficiency. When testosterone levels are below an average threshold of 12 nmol/L (346 ng/dL), testosterone replacement was shown to significantly increase libido and desire, the number of nocturnal erections, frequency of penetrative sex, International Index of Erectile Function (IIEF) scores, and overall sexual satisfaction in a 2005 meta-analysis. In men with ED and normal serum testosterone levels, however, there was no improvement in erectile function with testosterone therapy.[25] Other studies have shown contradictory data indicating that even eugonadal men may experience better erectile function with androgen therapy, thus calling into question the relationship between hypogonadism and ED.[26] Hyperprolactinemia is associated with sexual dysfunction and often ED, but this is likely a result of luteinizing hormone (LH) suppression and secondary hypogonadism. Hypothyroidism may also suppress LH secretion. Hyperthyroidism is associated with increased levels of serum estrogens. There is much debate and many ongoing investigations into the interplay between testosterone levels and erectile function.[27] Diabetes is a major cause of ED, not because of the short-term effects of impaired insulin secretion and hyperglycemia but because of the long-term damage to nerves and microvasculature; therefore, it is more accurately implicated in neurogenic and vasculogenic ED.

More than 200 medications, including entire drug classes, have been associated with ED. Approximately 25% of patients presenting with ED are taking offending medications, but often the underlying diseases treated by these medications are also associated with ED.[28] Antihypertensive agents are widely associated with ED, the most common offenders include β-blockers, clonidine, thiazide diuretics, angiotensin-converting enzyme inhibitors, and spironolactone. Essentially all classes of antidepressants (tricyclics, heterocyclics, selective serotonin reuptake inhibitors, and monoamine oxidase inhibitors) are notorious for their sexual side effects. Other psychiatric drugs associated with ED include benzodiazepines, antipsychotics, and phenytoin.[29] Risperidone and other typical antipsychotics like haloperidol and amisulpride block D_2 dopamine receptors and have a prolactin-elevating effect.[30] Other agents that may cause ED by lowering circulating testosterone levels include LH-releasing hormone agonists/antagonists, antiandrogens, and 5α-reductase inhibitors. Antiulcer drugs, opiates, and cytotoxic agents have also been associated with ED (**Table 1**).

Table 1 The A-list quick reference for some common causes of erectile dysfunction	
Psychogenic As	Anxiety, anhedonia (depression), adjustment disorder, adrenaline
Vasculogenic As	Arteriolosclerosis, arterial insufficiency, hemoglobin A_{1c}
Neurogenic As	Alzheimer, aging, hemoglobin A_{1c}, cvA, msA, acute trauma/infection
Endocrinologic As	Androgen deficiency, agonadal, hemoglobin A_{1c}
Pharmacologic As	Antidepressants, antihypertensives, anxiolytics, antipsychotics, antiandrogens, antiulcer, 5α-reductase inhibitors, alcohol, analgesic narcotics

Abbreviations: cvA, cerebrovascular accident; msA, multiple system atrophy.

EVALUATION: HISTORY

There are numerous reasons given by patients and clinicians alike for not discussing sexual history during an office visit. Patients often cite shame, embarrassment, lack of opportunity, and pessimism about the outcome of such a discussion as well as uncertainty about what is appropriate to address and with which doctor or specialty it should be addressed.[31] Clinicians are often concerned with time constraints, reimbursement, lack of knowledge/training, lack of available treatments, fear of offending patients, and discomfort in discussing sexual issues with those younger than 18, older than 65, or patients of the opposite gender.[31] In a survey of more than 27,000 patients, approximately half of the sexually active respondents, reported having at least 1 sexual problem, yet only 18% of those men attempted to seek medical help for these issues. Only 9% reported they had been asked about sexual health by a provider during a routine visit in the preceding 3 years.[32] It is universally acknowledged that sexual dysfunction, in particular ED, goes undiagnosed and undiscussed for a majority of men suffering its course. ED is not something that must be addressed at every clinical encounter, but it may be poignant to screen for sexual issues during annual visits, wellness checks, and when patients present with other neurologic, vascular, endocrine, or psychological symptoms. Certainly, if the topic is broached by the patient, even as an aside to the primary complaint, it warrants evaluation because it may weigh more heavily on the patient than he indicates and may be difficult for him to bring up again if it goes unaddressed.

First and foremost, before treating ED, a patient's cardiac risk should be assessed to ensure the heart is healthy enough to tolerate sexual activity. If considered high cardiac risk, then cardiology consultation should be pursued prior to treating ED. If at intermediate cardiac risk, then a cardiac stress test should be considered to better stratify into low risk versus high risk.[33] Patients who are asymptomatic with fewer than 3 major risk factors (hypertension, diabetes mellitus, cigarette smoking, dyslipidemia, sedentary lifestyle, and family history of premature coronary artery disease) are considered low risk and should proceed to comprehensive sexual history and treatment as indicated. Any modifiable risk factors identified in this process should be reviewed with the patient. Encouraging smoking cessation, control of blood sugar and blood pressure, increasing activity, and any other steps to optimize vascular health may improve erectile function and slow the inevitable age-related deterioration of erectile function as well as increase overall longevity.[34] The threat of complete and permanent loss of erectile function is often highly motivational for patients to improve their overall cardiovascular health and control diabetes.[35] In a survey asking impotent men with diabetes how much they would be willing to spend on treating complications from their diabetes, ED was ranked third behind renal failure and blindness.[35]

Once it is recognized that a patient self-identifies as having ED, it is first important to distinguish between ED and other common sexual dysfunctions, such as premature ejaculation, anejaculation, delayed orgasm, painful orgasm (dysorgasmia), lack of libido, Peyronie disease, and other penile deformities.[31] The formal definition of ED is fairly subjective: the inability to achieve and/or maintain erection of sufficient rigidity and duration to permit satisfactory sexual performance. Therefore, making a diagnosis is fairly straightforward based on a reliable patient history alone. A complete history should include onset, duration, rigidity with a partner, rigidity with masturbation, ability to penetrate, ability to sustain the erection, presence and quality of nocturnal erections, and prior ED treatments used and their efficacies.[31] A thorough surgical history, specifically asking about any previous abdominal, pelvic, penile, or scrotal surgeries, should identify patients at risk of vascular insufficiency secondary to surgical trauma as well as patients who may have corporal denervation after radical prostatectomy, cystectomy, colorectal surgery, or exenteration of other pelvic organs.[36–38] Teasing out the specific subtype of ED for each patient can be difficult if not impossible, because many patients have a multifactorial etiology, as previously discussed. In the end, determining the exact cause of a patient's ED may be helpful for treating underlying conditions and for guiding more advanced treatments but is usually unnecessary before initiating first-line therapies because nearly all types of ED are treated similarly and in a stepwise fashion.

In determining the presence and degree of ED and monitoring progress and effectiveness of treatment, it is often helpful to have a patient fill out a self-reported survey. There are several validated questionnaires used in sexual medicine practice to identify and quantify the degree of ED.[39] The IIEF, introduced in 1997, was originally developed for use in the clinical trials evaluating sildenafil as a treatment of ED. It is now recognized as the gold standard instrument for measuring efficacy in clinical trials for ED interventions.[40] The IIEF has been validated in 32 languages and consists of 15 self-administered questions addressing the domains of male sexual function, including erectile function, orgasmic function, sexual desire, intercourse satisfaction, and overall satisfaction.[41] An abridged version, known as the IIEF-5, takes only 5 questions from the IIEF and has become the preferred tool for evaluating ED for many providers for its ease of administration and validated specificity for ED. Each question is scored on a scale from 1 to 5, with a score of 5 generally indicating optimal performance and 1 indicating the highest degree of dysfunction. The sum of the 5 scores then stratifies a patient's level of ED from "severe ED" to "no ED" (**Table 2**).

The Sexual Health Inventory for Men (SHIM) is often referred to interchangeably as the IIEF-5. The only difference between the 2 is that some versions of the SHIM questionnaire allow for a score of 0 on 4 of the questions to indicate either "no sexual activity" or "did not attempt intercourse" resulting in the severe ED category expanded to a range of 1 to 7.[42] To further simplify the process, it has been suggested that a single-question screening tool may be useful in identifying patients with ED. A subset of 137 male patients ages 55 to 85 from the MMAS were screened with the single question, asking them to characterize their ability to "get and keep an erection good enough for sexual intercourse" as either "always," "usually," "sometimes," or "never." Patients were then evaluated with a full urologic examination, developed by the Process of Care Consensus Panel for ED,[43] to obtain a clinical diagnosis of ED. The 75.2% of patients identified as having ED by the single-question method was nearly identical to the 75.9% determined to have ED by urologic examination. The stratification of ED into severity categories was not as strongly correlated, but by using "minimal" as the cut-point for self-reported ED, the researchers found the single-question tool to have a sensitivity of 91% and specificity of approximately 76%, making the diagnosis of clinical ED with "reasonable accuracy."[44]

Table 2 International index of erectile function –5 questionnaire	
Score on International Index of Erectile Function –5 Questionnaire	Degree of Erectile Dysfunction
22–25	No ED
17–21	Mild ED
12–16	Mild to moderate ED
8–11	Moderate ED
5–7	Severe ED

The Erection Hardness Score is another single-item Likert scale that was also developed to evaluate effectiveness of sildenafil but has since been applied to and validated for[45] other treatments as well, including intracavernosal prostaglandins (**Table 3**).[46]

EVALUATION: PHYSICAL EXAMINATION

A patient's vital signs may be the first indicator of a precipitating condition in an ED patient. Look for evidence of hypertension, cardiac arrhythmia, weak pulse, tachycardia, or bradycardia. If suspicious features are noted, a more complete vascular examination may be warranted, including palpation of abdominal aorta for aneurysm and palpation of peripheral pulses.[47] Waist circumference and BMI, both independent risk factors for ED, should be measured and addressed.[48] Look for signs of androgen deficiency: gynecomastia, beard growth, pubic hair, testicular size and location, phallus length, and girth. The genitourinary examination should also include thorough palpation of the entire length of penile shaft for deformities, scars, Peyronie plaques, and location of the urethral meatus. Size and character of the prostate and seminal vesicles may be evaluated with digital rectal examination because concomitant prostate pathology is often noted in patients presenting with ED. Ultimately, the physical examination may not elucidate the exact cause of the ED, but it should help identify any underlying sexual or urologic abnormalities, and it may lead to the diagnosis of other urgent or even life-threatening comorbidities.[47]

EVALUATION: LABORATORY VALUES AND OTHER TESTS

Laboratory testing is not necessary in every patient with ED, although it may reveal underlying pathology associated with ED, especially in patients who have not been followed regularly by a primary care provider. To look for underlying cardiovascular risk, serum fasting lipids and fasting glucose or hemoglobin A_{1c} are helpful. Testosterone levels may be checked for those men with ED and low libido, decreased energy, increased fatigability, or other signs/symptoms of hypogonadism. Serum testosterone is typically checked in the early morning because it tends to be highest at this time and decrease throughout the day at least in younger men. When testosterone is found to be low, a prolactin level is helpful in differentiating between primary hypogonadism and testosterone suppression secondary to a prolactin-secreting pituitary microadenoma. PSA testing may be discussed with patients over age 40 to 45 particularly if a patient will be receiving supplemental testosterone. Thyroid testing is another consideration depending on patient presentation and clinical picture.[47]

In addition to serum testing, there are several investigational studies that can be conducted to help determine ED etiology. Most of these investigations have limited utility in clinical practice because there is little evidence to suggest they alter patient management. Biothesiometry is an assessment of penile vibratory sensation where a stimulator is first applied at very low intensity and then gradually increased until

Table 3	
Erection hardness score	
Erection Hardness Scale	**Patient Response**
0	Penis does not enlarge
1	Penis is larger but not hard
2	Penis is hard but not hard enough for penetration
3	Penis is hard enough for penetration but not completely hard
4	Penis is completely hard and fully rigid

the patient reports the first sensation. The lower this threshold for sensation, the greater the neural integrity is thought to be. If the penile threshold is significantly lower than for other areas of the body, this is considered a positive screen for penile neuropathy.[49] Pudendal somatosensory evoked potentials, performed by neurologists or other specialists, aim to evaluate afferent sensory spinal pathways by measuring latency time of electrical stimulus from penis to brain.[50]

Vascular testing for ED can be used to assess the vascular integrity of the corpora cavernosa and to potentially identify patients with inadequate veno-occlusive function, termed *venous leak*. One simple test, often performed as part of an injection therapy teaching visit, is to inject the corpora with a vasoactive agent, such as alprostadil, papaverine, or other erectogenic drug. If an adequate erection is achieved after approximately 10 minutes, then vascular insufficiency is unlikely. If the erection is maintained, then venous leak is not a factor. Inability to achieve an erection or early loss of the erection after injection, however, is not diagnostic of vascular insufficiency or venous leakage. Penile duplex Doppler ultrasound (DDUS) can be performed after injection of vasoactive erectogenic drugs to measure intracavernosal peak systolic velocity at maximal erection as well as end-diastolic velocity. Peak systolic velocity less than 30 cm/s supports a diagnosis of arterial insufficiency, and end-diastolic velocity greater than 5 cm/s suggests venous leak. DDUS does not necessarily change the treatment plan, but it may be useful to rule out organic pathology in patients with purely psychogenic ED, and it may encourage other men to seek definitive surgical management with penile prosthesis if it confirms that even with maximal pharmacotherapy, the penile vasculature simply will not support satisfactory rigidity.[51] More invasive studies, such as cavernosometry and cavernosography, are more accurate in diagnosing venous leak but are rarely used in the modern era. Pudendal angiography may be used in patients who have diagnosed arterial insufficiency by DDUS or cavernosometry and plan to undergo revascularization surgery.[52]

MANAGEMENT

ED is typically treated in a stepwise fashion, often irrespective of etiology. In terms of preventing further or progressive blood flow impedance and/or neurologic damage, however, it is of upmost importance to identify and treat modifiable risk factors and comorbidities, such as diabetes, hypertension, hyperlipidemia, CAD, systemic inflammatory disorders, and so forth. The MMAS data suggest that lifestyle changes targeting modifiable risk factors, such as smoking, heavy alcohol consumption, sedentary lifestyle, and obesity, are most effective when started before age 50.[53] First-line medical therapy usually consists of a trial of oral phosphodiesterase type 5 inhibitors (PDE5Is). Failure of a PDE5I usually precedes a trial of another PDE5I because some patients may respond better to one agent over another or may find the dosing and timing requirements easier to follow for a particular drug. Second-line therapies include intracavernosal injection therapy, intraurethral suppositories, and vacuum erection devices (VEDs). Third-line management involves surgical intervention.

Phosphodiesterase Type 5 Inhibitors

PDE is the enzyme that degrades cGMP and leads to increased smooth muscle tone and decreased cavernosal blood flow. PDE5Is, therefore, prolong the action of cGMP created during sexual stimulation leading to more rigidity and longer duration of erections. Of these agents, sildenafil has the longest history of utilization in ED and is also the most widely studied. Other agents have been developed to alter the time of onset, duration of action and other pharmacokinetic factors. Sildenafil is dosed approximately 1 hour prior to sexual activity, has an oral bioavailability of 41%, has elimination half-life of 4 hours, and has better absorption on an empty stomach because the effect of food may delay time to maximum plasma concentration (T_{max}) by 60 minutes and reduce maximum serum concentration by 29% (Micromedex). It is supplied in 25-mg, 50-mg, and 100-mg tablets. Tadalafil reaches Tmax at 2 to 4 hours and absorption is not affected by food. Elimination half-life is much longer at 15 hours to 35 hours and, therefore, is many times preferred by patients who desire more spontaneity or have a harder time planning their sexual activity. Tadalafil may be dosed as 10 mg to 20 mg on demand like sildenafil, or it may be taken as a 2.5-mg to 5-mg daily dose to achieve a reasonable steady-state concentration allowing for maximum spontaneity. A systematic review and meta-analysis published in 2013 concluded that PDE5 inhibitors, in recommended doses, are more effective than placebo for ED, and that PDE5Is are generally safe and well tolerated without any major differences in safety profiles.[54] PDE5Is are contraindicated in patients who take daily nitrates and should be used with extreme caution in any patients who have access to nitrates but do not use them regularly, such as nitroglycerin for angina. Combining PDE5Is with nitrates may lead to sudden and life-threatening hypotension. Extra attention should be given to patients who take α-blockers for hypertension or BPH because there is some evidence this may worsen orthostatic symptoms, and it is generally suggested to start at the lowest dose before titrating up as tolerated. Vardenafil should be avoided in patients with congenital QT syndrome and in those taking type 1A or type 3 antiarrhythmics. PDE5I are metabolized via the cytochrome CYP3A4 pathway. Other drugs also metabolized by CYP3A4 include antiretroviral protease inhibitors, azole antifungals, and macrolide antibiotics.[55] Common adverse effects of PDE5Is include headache, flushing, nasal congestion, heartburn, muscle aches, and vision changes.[54] Patients should always be cautioned about priapism and instructed to seek medical attention for erections lasting longer than 4 hours, although there are only a handful of reported cases of priapism from PDE5Is alone in patients without any underlying conditions predisposing them to priapism (sickle cell disease or trait, thrombocytopenia, multiple myeloma, and polycythemia) (**Table 4**).[56]

Table 4
Phosphodiesterase type 5 inhibitors dosing

Phosphodiesterase Type 5 Inhibitors	Trade Name and Date Approved	Doses Supplied	Timing Relative to Intercourse	Onset	Half-Life	Meal Timing
Sildenafil	Viagra, 1998	25 mg, 50 mg, 100 mg	60 min	14–60 min	4 h	Take on empty stomach
Tadalafil	Cialis, 2003	2.5 mg, 5 mg, 10 mg, 20 mg	1–12 h	16–45 min	17.5 h	Not affected by meals
Vardenafil	Levitra, 2003	5 mg, 10 mg, 20 mg	60 min	25 min	4–5 h	Decreased effect
Vardenafil ODT	Staxyn, 2010	10 mg	90 min	—	4–6 h	Decreased effect
Avanafil	Stendra, 2012	100 mg, 200 mg	30 min	30–45 min	5 h	Decreased effect

From Smith-Harrison LI, Patel A, Smith RP. The devil is in the details: an analysis of the subtleties between phosphodiesterase inhibitors for erectile dysfunction. Transl Androl Urol 2016;5(2):181–6.

Vacuum Erection Device

A VED is considered second-line therapy for ED after failure of PDE5I or when upstream damage to the cGMP/NO pathway from damage to the cavernosal nerve (radical prostatectomy or autonomic diabetic neuropathy) renders PDE5I ineffective. Although there are many different models of VED, the set-up generally includes a cylinder that can be placed over the shaft of the penis and held to form an air-tight seal against the body; a pump mechanism evacuates air from the cylinder, thus creating a negative pressure around the penile shaft, promoting cavernosal filling with venous blood; and a constriction band that can be slipped off of the proximal end of the cylinder onto the base of the penis to maintain penile tumescence after the cylinder is removed. The band should be removed within 30 minutes to avoid ecchymosis and skin necrosis. Barriers to patient use may include inability to make an adequate seal against the skin, painful ejaculation secondary to urethral compression from the constriction band, a darker/cooler erection from venous filling rather than arterial, and poor manual dexterity. Many of the medical-grade devices come with helpful instruction manuals and videos for teaching and often the companies offer one-on-one teaching with a device representative who may meet with patients in a physician's office setting when allowed.[57,58]

Intraurethral Suppositories

Prostaglandin E1 (PGE1) is a direct stimulator of intracellular cAMP in smooth muscle, initiating a cascade that leads to sequestration of intracellular calcium resulting in cavernosal smooth muscle relaxation and penile erection.[59] PGE1 can be delivered as a small suppository inserted into the urethra through the meatus. The penile shaft is then massaged and rolled between the hands to promote dissolving and absorption of the suppository across the corpus spongiosum and into the corpora cavernosa through collateral vessels. Penile pain is a common side effect along with urethral burning. Priapism is a rare but documented risk. A test dose is typically administered under medical supervision to ensure the patient will tolerate the medication and to look for symptomatic hypotension seen in as high as 2% of patients at maximum dosage.

Intracavernosal Injections

Intracavernosal injections (ICIs) for ED actually predate use of oral PDE5I yet are still widely regarded as one of the safest and most effective treatments for ED.[60] Similar to intraurethral suppositories, PGE1 is the most common agent used in ICI therapy. There are proprietary forms of injectable PGE1 available at various concentrations in both prefilled syringes and in vials of powder for reconstitution. Alternatively, sterile compounding pharmacies often formulate their own compounded PGE1 for injection and have the ability to combine it with other erectogenic agents, such as papaverine and phentolamine, to create what is commonly known as bimix or trimix. Papaverine inhibits PDEs nonspecifically to increase intracellular concentrations of both cAMP and cGMP and promote smooth muscle relaxation. Phentolamine inhibits α_1-adrenergic receptors effectively blocking vasoconstriction by reducing sympathetic tone. Although there are no specific guidelines as to which doses and concentrations are to be used, it is generally best to start with a low dose and slowly titrate up over several days or weeks until an optimal erection is achieved. A test dose in the office is helpful to teach patients how to select and draw up their dose, how to locate the corpora cavernosa, and how to inject intracavernosally while avoiding important structures, such as the urethra, the dorsal veins and nerves, and any prominent superficial veins that may cause bruising or hematoma.[61] Optimally, a patient injects the dorsolateral aspect of the base to midpenile shaft on one side, and the site of injection is varied with each dose to prevent scarring. It is not recommended to exceed 1 dose in 24 hours or to dose more frequently than 3 times per week because more frequent dosing may theoretically increase risk of priapism or scarring and fibrosis. Barriers to patient compliance with ICIs include anxiety, fear of needles, stinging at the injection site, and pain or aching from the erectogenic drugs, most commonly PGE1, with up to 50% of men reporting some degree of discomfort, especially those with a history of pelvic surgery.[62] Patients may increase their injected volumes and report back progress. If a large volume fails to produce an adequate erection, then a new formulation with a higher concentration and/or addition of other agents may be prescribed. If a high-volume of high-concentration trimix fails to produce an erection, then it is often time to consider surgical management of ED.

Penile Implant Surgery

Third-line therapy for ED involves surgical placement of a penile prosthesis. Penile implants are broadly categorized into noninflatable implants, 2-piece inflatable implants, and 3-piece inflatable implants.[63]

Noninflatable or malleable implants are flexible rods inserted into each corporal body. The cylindrical rods can then be bent downward when not in use or bent upward to straighten the penile shaft and simulate and erection. There is no flaccid state with a malleable implant, so more caution must be exercised in patients with loss of sensation to ensure the constant pressure of the device does not result in erosion through the distal glans.

A 2-piece inflatable penile prosthesis (IPP) includes 2 inflatable cylinders within the corpora connected to a small pump hidden in the scrotum. When in the flaccid state, the fluid resides in the more proximal base of the cylinders. The scrotal pump is then depressed multiple times to transfer fluid from the proximal reservoir into the decompressed distal portion of the cylinders. The IPP is delated by bending the cylinders to a 90° angle, which then transfers fluid back to the proximal reservoir. The 2-piece IPP is primarily used in patients for whom placement of a separate fluid reservoir intra-abdominally is difficult, dangerous, or impossible.

A 3-piece IPP consists also of 2 inflatable cylinders in the corpora. The pump in the scrotum has a compressible end for inflation as well as a button or separate mechanism to open a valve allowing flow of fluid from the cylinders back to the reservoir for deflation. In the 3-piece IPP, the reservoir is a separate balloon that is traditionally placed intra-abdominally through the inguinal ring in the space of Retzius; however, more modern techniques have demonstrated safe placement of the reservoir in ectopic locations, such as in a submsuclular tunnel developed between the peritoneum and transversalis fascia, deep to the rectus abdominis.

Candidates for IPP should have good manual dexterity and sensation to allow for locating the pump among the other scrotal contents and to ensure ability to squeeze the pump with adequate force while stabilizing the pump to prevent it slipping painfully out of grip.

Although mechanical failure is always a possibility (5%–10% after 10 years),[64] the most severe and devastating complication is infection, because the device must be completely explanted, with tissue washout and systemic antibiotics, and traditionally a 3-month waiting period before another implant can be attempted. Infections are more common with longer surgical times or less-experienced implanters and in patients with diabetes, especially poorly controlled (hemoglobin A_{1c} >8).

It is important to manage patient expectations before implant surgery. No matter how much care is taken to maximize length and ensure that cylinders fit the native corporal size, there nearly always is some perception of loss of length and/or girth with erection and a decrease or absence of the natural lengthening of the shaft some men experience during tumescence. Ideally the device provides excellent rigidity for reliable on-demand erections, but it will certainly not look and feel as natural as patients remember from their youth.

SUMMARY

Over the past 25 years, ED has gone from a vague, underdiagnosed, difficult-to-treat disease process to a clearly defined pathologic state with well described though complex etiologies, a variety of tools for screening and evaluation, and an explosion of treatment options that provide clinicians a logical, stepwise algorithm to help patients restore erectile function and reclaim their sexual health. As the taboo around sexual dysfunction has diminished, ED has been recognized by general practitioners and cardiologists as an important risk factor for microvascular disease and a potential harbinger of cardiovascular disease. As the field of ED treatment has expanded, new pharmacologic agents have continued to be developed, new strategies such as extracorporeal shockwave therapy have been explored, and surgical techniques and prosthetics have been constantly revised and refined. In essence the modern study and treatment of ED are still burgeoning frontiers in the fight against an ancient disease.

REFERENCES

1. Shokeir AA, Hussein MI. Sexual life in pharaonic Egypt: towards a urological view. Int J Impot Res 2004;16(5):385–8.
2. Impotence. NIH Consensus Statement 1992;10(4):1–33.
3. Feldman HA, Goldstein I, Hatzichristou DG, et al. Impotence and its medical and psychosocial correlates: results of the Massachusetts male aging study. J Urol 1994;151(1):54–61.
4. Brookes ST, Link CL, Donovan JL, et al. Relationship between lower urinary tract symptoms and erectile dysfunction: results from the Boston area community health survey. J Urol 2008;179(1):250–5 [discussion: 255].
5. Laumann EO, Nicolosi A, Glasser DB, et al. Sexual problems among women and men aged 40-80 y: prevalence and correlates identified in the global study of sexual attitudes and behaviors. Int J Impotence Res 2005;17(1):39–57.
6. Skrypnik D, Bogdanski P, Musialik K. Obesity–significant risk factor for erectile dysfunction in men. Polski Merkuriusz Lekarski 2014;36(212):137–41 [in Polish].
7. Sommer F, Goldstein I, Korda JB. Bicycle riding and erectile dysfunction: a review. J Sex Med 2010;7(7):2346–58.
8. Bacon CG, Mittleman MA, Kawachi I, et al. A prospective study of risk factors for erectile dysfunction. J Urol 2006;176(1):217–21.
9. Jeon YJ, Yoon DW, Han DH, et al. Low quality of life and depressive symptoms as an independent risk factor for erectile dysfunction in patients with obstructive sleep apnea. J Sex Med 2015;12(11):2168–77.
10. Sanjay S, Bharti GS, Manish G, et al. Metabolic syndrome: an independent risk factor for erectile dysfunction. Indian J Endocrinol Metab 2015;19(2):277–82.

11. Kalka D, Domagala Z, Rakowska A, et al. Modifiable risk factors for erectile dysfunction: an assessment of the awareness of such factors in patients suffering from ischaemic heart disease. Int J Impotence Res 2016;28(1):14–9.

12. El-Assmy A, Harraz AM, Benhassan M, et al. Erectile dysfunction post-perineal anastomotic urethroplasty for traumatic urethral injuries: analysis of incidence and possibility of recovery. Int Urol Nephrol 2015;47(5):797–802.

13. Breza J, Aboseif SR, Orvis BR, et al. Detailed anatomy of penile neurovascular structures: surgical significance. J Urol 1989;141(2):437–43.

14. Lue TF, Tanagho EA. Physiology of erection and pharmacological management of impotence. J Urol 1987;137(5):829–36.

15. Yang CC, Jiang X. Clinical autonomic neurophysiology and the male sexual response: an overview. J Sex Med 2009;6(Suppl 3):221–8.

16. Prieto D. Physiological regulation of penile arteries and veins. Int J Impotence Res 2008;20(1):17–29.

17. Lue TF, Takamura T, Schmidt RA, et al. Hemodynamics of erection in the monkey. J Urol 1983;130(6):1237–41.

18. Melman A, Gingell JC. The epidemiology and pathophysiology of erectile dysfunction. J Urol 1999;161(1):5–11.

19. Trussell JC, Kunselman AR, Legro RS. Epinephrine is associated with both erectile dysfunction and lower urinary tract symptoms. Fertil Sterility 2010;93(3): 837–42.

20. Liu C, Lu K, Tao T, et al. Endothelial nitric oxide synthase polymorphisms and erectile dysfunction: a meta-analysis. J Sex Med 2015;12(6):1319–28.

21. Muniz JJ, Lacchini R, Rinaldi TO, et al. Endothelial nitric oxide synthase genotypes and haplotypes modify the responses to sildenafil in patients with erectile dysfunction. Pharmacogenomics J Apr 2013;13(2):189–96.

22. Soni SD, Song W, West JL, et al. Nitric oxide-releasing polymeric microspheres improve diabetes-related erectile dysfunction. J Sex Med 2013;10(8):1915–25.

23. Burnett AL. The role of nitric oxide in erectile dysfunction: implications for medical therapy. J Clin Hypertens 2006;8(12 Suppl 4):53–62.

24. Winder K, Seifert F, Kohrmann M, et al. Lesion mapping of stroke-related erectile dysfunction. Brain 2017;140(6):1706–17.

25. Isidori AM, Giannetta E, Gianfrilli D, et al. Effects of testosterone on sexual function in men: results of a meta-analysis. Clin Endocrinol 2005;63(4):381–94.

26. Buvat J, Lemaire A. Endocrine screening in 1,022 men with erectile dysfunction: clinical significance and cost-effective strategy. J Urol 1997;158(5):1764–7.

27. Bhasin S, Enzlin P, Coviello A, et al. Sexual dysfunction in men and women with endocrine disorders. Lancet 2007;369(9561):597–611.

28. Keene LC, Davies PH. Drug-related erectile dysfunction. Adverse Drug React Toxicol Rev 1999;18(1):5–24.

29. Francis ME, Kusek JW, Nyberg LM, et al. The contribution of common medical conditions and drug exposures to erectile dysfunction in adult males. J Urol 2007;178(2):591–6 [discussion: 596].

30. Park YW, Kim Y, Lee JH. Antipsychotic-induced sexual dysfunction and its management. World J Mens Health 2012;30(3):153–9.

31. Althof SE, Rosen RC, Perelman MA, et al. Standard operating procedures for taking a sexual history. J Sex Med 2013;10(1):26–35.

32. Moreira ED Jr, Brock G, Glasser DB, et al. Help-seeking behaviour for sexual problems: the global study of sexual attitudes and behaviors. Int J Clin Pract 2005;59(1):6–16.

33. Kostis JB, Jackson G, Rosen R, et al. Sexual dysfunction and cardiac risk (the Second Princeton Consensus Conference). Am J Cardiol 2005;96(12B):85M–93M.
34. Gupta BP, Murad MH, Clifton MM, et al. The effect of lifestyle modification and cardiovascular risk factor reduction on erectile dysfunction: a systematic review and meta-analysis. Arch Intern Med 2011;171(20):1797–803.
35. Rance J, Phillips C, Davies S, et al. How much of a priority is treating erectile dysfunction? A study of patients' perceptions. Diabetic Med 2003;20(3):205–9.
36. Celentano V, Cohen R, Warusavitarne J, et al. Sexual dysfunction following rectal cancer surgery. Int J Colorectal Dis 2017. [Epub ahead of print].
37. Bratu O, Oprea I, Marcu D, et al. Erectile dysfunction post-radical prostatectomy - a challenge for both patient and physician. J Med Life 2017;10(1):13–8.
38. Nandipati KC, Raina R, Agarwal A, et al. Erectile dysfunction following radical retropubic prostatectomy: epidemiology, pathophysiology and pharmacological management. Drugs Aging 2006;23(2):101–17.
39. Giuliano F. Questionnaires in sexual medicine. Prog Urol 2013;23(9):811–21 [in French].
40. Rosen RC, Cappelleri JC, Gendrano N 3rd. The International Index of Erectile Function (IIEF): a state-of-the-science review. Int J Impotence Res 2002;14(4):226–44.
41. Rosen RC, Riley A, Wagner G, et al. The international index of erectile function (IIEF): a multidimensional scale for assessment of erectile dysfunction. Urology 1997;49(6):822–30.
42. Cappelleri JC, Rosen RC. The Sexual Health Inventory for Men (SHIM): a 5-year review of research and clinical experience. Int J impotence Res 2005;17(4):307–19.
43. The process of care model for evaluation and treatment of erectile dysfunction. The process of care consensus panel. Int J Impotence Res 1999;11(2):59–70 [discussion: 70–54].
44. O'Donnell AB, Araujo AB, Goldstein I, et al. The validity of a single-question self-report of erectile dysfunction. results from the Massachusetts male aging study. J Gen Intern Med 2005;20(6):515–9.
45. Mulhall JP, Goldstein I, Bushmakin AG, et al. Validation of the erection hardness score. J Sex Med 2007;4(6):1626–34.
46. Parisot J, Yiou R, Salomon L, et al. Erection hardness score for the evaluation of erectile dysfunction: further psychometric assessment in patients treated by intracavernous prostaglandins injections after radical prostatectomy. J Sex Med 2014;11(8):2109–18.
47. Ghanem HM, Salonia A, Martin-Morales A. SOP: physical examination and laboratory testing for men with erectile dysfunction. J Sex Med 2013;10(1):108–10.
48. Walls HL, Stevenson CE, Mannan HR, et al. Comparing trends in BMI and waist circumference. Obesity 2011;19(1):216–9.
49. Bemelmans BL, Hendrikx LB, Koldewijn EL, et al. Comparison of biothesiometry and neuro-urophysiological investigations for the clinical evaluation of patients with erectile dysfunction. J Urol 1995;153(5):1483–6.
50. Giuliano F, Rowland DL. Standard operating procedures for neurophysiologic assessment of male sexual dysfunction. J Sex Med 2013;10(5):1205–11.
51. Sikka SC, Hellstrom WJ, Brock G, et al. Standardization of vascular assessment of erectile dysfunction: standard operating procedures for duplex ultrasound. J Sex Med 2013;10(1):120–9.

52. Spiliopoulos S, Shaida N, Katsanos K, et al. The role of interventional radiology in the diagnosis and management of male impotence. Cardiovasc Interv Radiol 2013;36(5):1204–12.
53. Derby CA, Mohr BA, Goldstein I, et al. Modifiable risk factors and erectile dysfunction: can lifestyle changes modify risk? Urology 2000;56(2):302–6.
54. Yuan J, Zhang R, Yang Z, et al. Comparative effectiveness and safety of oral phosphodiesterase type 5 inhibitors for erectile dysfunction: a systematic review and network meta-analysis. Eur Urol 2013;63(5):902–12.
55. Corona G, Razzoli E, Forti G, et al. The use of phosphodiesterase 5 inhibitors with concomitant medications. J Endocrinological Invest 2008;31(9):799–808.
56. McMahon CG. Priapism associated with concurrent use of phosphodiesterase inhibitor drugs and intracavernous injection therapy. Int J Impotence Res 2003; 15(5):383–4.
57. Ganem JP, Lucey DT, Janosko EO, et al. Unusual complications of the vacuum erection device. Urology 1998;51(4):627–31.
58. Baltaci S, Aydos K, Kosar A, et al. Treating erectile dysfunction with a vacuum tumescence device: a retrospective analysis of acceptance and satisfaction. Br J Urol 1995;76(6):757–60.
59. Palmer LS, Valcic M, Melman A, et al. Characterization of cyclic AMP accumulation in cultured human corpus cavernosum smooth muscle cells. J Urol 1994; 152(4):1308–14.
60. Shabsigh R, Padma-Nathan H, Gittleman M, et al. Intracavernous alprostadil alfadex (EDEX/VIRIDAL) is effective and safe in patients with erectile dysfunction after failing sildenafil (Viagra). Urology 2000;55(4):477–80.
61. Hsiao W, Bennett N, Guhring P, et al. Satisfaction profiles in men using intracavernosal injection therapy. J Sex Med 2011;8(2):512–7.
62. Nelson CJ, Hsiao W, Balk E, et al. Injection anxiety and pain in men using intracavernosal injection therapy after radical pelvic surgery. J Sex Med 2013;10(10): 2559–65.
63. Minervini A, Ralph DJ, Pryor JP. Outcome of penile prosthesis implantation for treating erectile dysfunction: experience with 504 procedures. BJU Int 2006; 97(1):129–33.
64. Holloway FB, Farah RN. Intermediate term assessment of the reliability, function and patient satisfaction with the AMS700 ultrex penile prosthesis. J Urol 1997; 157(5):1687–91.

Hypogonadism
Evaluation Management and Treatment Considerations

Kenneth A. Mitchell, MPAS, PA-C

KEYWORDS

- Hypogonadism • Testosterone replacement therapy • Metabolic syndrome
- Prostate cancer • Physician assistant

KEY POINTS

- There is an increase in the prevalence of hypogonadism in both younger and older men.
- The evaluation of men with hypogonadism is often poorly understood, leading to suboptimal treatment.
- Hypogonadism has been shown to be associated with cardiometabolic disease and, therefore, requires a thorough evaluation that addresses the various associated comorbidities.
- Controversies related to the treatment of hypogonadism in men with prostate cancer remains a topic of much debate.
- Large randomized controlled trials will need to be conducted to provide clinicians with the most accurate evidence regarding the safety of testosterone replacement therapy (TRT) and the impact of TRT on alleviating or controlling associated comorbidities.

INTRODUCTION

Hypogonadism, also referred to as testosterone deficiency, is defined as a decrease in the concentration of serum total testosterone (<300 ng/dL) and/or a decrease in sperm production.[1] Signs and symptoms include decreased libido, fatigue, erectile dysfunction, loss of body and facial hair, decreased bone mineral density, increased body fat, decreased lean muscle mass, weakness, depressed mood, sleep disturbance, and anemia. The prevalence of hypogonadism in men aged 45 years or older visiting primary care practices in the United States is estimated to be approximately 38.7%.[2] Further evidence indicates there is a higher prevalence of hypogonadism in men with obesity, diabetes, hypertension, rheumatoid arthritis, hyperlipidemia, and osteopenia or osteoporosis.[2] Conflicting evidence on the prevalence of hypogonadism

---

Disclosures: The author has nothing to disclose.
Meharry Medical College Physician Assistant Sciences Program, Meharry Medical College, 1005 Dr D. B. Todd Jr. Boulevard, Nashville, TN 37208, USA
E-mail address: kmitchell@mmc.edu

Physician Assist Clin 3 (2018) 129–137
http://dx.doi.org/10.1016/j.cpha.2017.08.009
2405-7991/18/© 2017 Elsevier Inc. All rights reserved.

physicianassistant.theclinics.com

combined with the constellation of symptoms can lead to suboptimal evaluations of men presenting with testosterone deficiency. Most clinicians follow the guidelines established by the Endocrine Society; however, the American Association of Clinical Endocrinologists Guidelines, and the *International Society for Sexual Medicine's Process of Care for the Assessment and Management of Testosterone Deficiency in Adult Men* can make it difficult to reach a consensus on the best practice approach for the evaluation, treatment, and management of hypogonadism in men.[3]

EVALUATION OF HYPOGONADISM

Initial evaluation of men with hypogonadism presenting with 1 or more objective symptoms (**Table 1**) should begin with a comprehensive history and identification of potential comorbidities associated with hypogonadism (**Table 2**). A thorough physical examination should include identifying the presence of gynecomastia, the presence of secondary sex characteristics (decreased body hair [pubic or axillary], decreased beard growth), a testicular examination paying close attention to the size and consistency of the testicles (adult testes are usually between 20 and 30 mL in volume and from 4.5 to 6.5 cm long by 2.8–3.3 cm wide), prostate examination, and body mass index (BMI).[1,4] Laboratory testing parameters vary between the published guidelines; however, all agree that measurement of a morning total testosterone level by a reliable assay and confirmed by repeat measurement should be obtained to confirm the diagnosis. Men with total testosterone near the lower limit of normal or in men in whom sex hormone-binding globulin abnormality is suspected (eg, older men, men with obesity, diabetes mellitus, chronic illness, liver disease, or thyroid disease) should have additional laboratory testing performed (**Table 3**). Further laboratory testing should include serum luteinizing hormone (LH) and follicle-stimulating hormone (FSH) levels to distinguish between primary (testicular) and secondary (pituitary-hypothalamic) hypogonadism. Measurement of LH and FSH concentrations can help distinguish between primary and secondary hypogonadism. Men with primary hypogonadism have low testosterone levels with elevated LH and FSH levels, whereas men with secondary hypogonadism have low testosterone levels with low or normal LH levels. Serum LH levels in men with secondary hypogonadism may be below the normal range or in the low-normal range but clearly inappropriate in relation to the low testosterone

Table 1 Clinical presentation of hypogonadism		
Physical	**Psychological**	**Sexual**
Decreased bone mineral density	Diminished energy, sense of vitality, or well-being	Decrease spontaneous directions
Decrease muscle mass and strength	Impaired cognition and memory	Erectile dysfunction
Gynecomastia	Decreased mood	Difficulty achieving orgasm
Anemia Frailty Increased body mass index Fatigue Insulin resistance Enlarged liver or elevated liver function tests		Diminished libido

Data from Refs.[1,4,5]

Table 2
Prevalence rates and odds ratios for selected risk factors in enrolled untreated hypogonadal patients

Risk Factor or Condition	Hypogonadism Prevalence Rate (95% CI)	Odds Ratio (95% CI)
Obesity	52.4 (47.9–56.9)	2.38 (1.93–2.93)
Diabetes	50.0 (45.5–54.5)	2.09 (1.70–2.58)
Hypertension	42.4 (39.6–45.2)	1.84 (1.53–2.22)
Rheumatoid arthritis	47.3 (34.1–60.5)	1.59 (0.92–2.72)
Hyperlipidemia	40.4 (37.6–43.3)	1.47 (1.23–1.76)
Osteoporosis	44.4 (25.5–64.7)	1.41 (0.64–3.01)
Asthma or COPD	43.5 (36.8–50.3)	1.40 (1.04–1.86)
Prostatic disease or disorder	41.3 (36.4–46.2)	1.29 (1.03–1.62)
Chronic pain	38.8 (33.7–44.0)	1.13 (0.89–1.44)
Headaches (within last 2 wk)	32.1 (25.3–38.8)	0.81 (0.58–1.11)

Abbreviations: CI, confidence interval; COPD, chronic obstructive pulmonary disease.
From Mulligan T, Frick M, Zuraw Q, et al. Prevalence of hypogonadism in males aged at least 45 years: the HIM study. Int J Clin Pract 2006;60(7):766; with permission.

concentrations. In patients in whom secondary hypogonadism is suspected, further evaluation should include measurements of serum prolactin, pituitary function testing, and MRI of the pituitary gland. In men with primary testicular failure of unknown cause and a physical examination yielding low testicular volume and lack of secondary sexual characteristics, obtaining a karyotype to exclude Klinefelter syndrome (XXY male) is recommended. Men with Klinefelter syndrome can benefit from genetic counseling and need surveillance for certain disorders for which they are at increased risk.[6] In men being evaluated for infertility, the Endocrine Society guidelines and the American Urological Association (AUA) publication, The Optimal Evaluation of the Infertile Male: AUA Best Practice Statement both recommend obtaining at least 2 semen analyses separated by an interval of several weeks. The sample should be evaluated within 1 hour of ejaculation and after at least 48 hours of abstinence for consideration with the patient's hormonal data.[1,7,8] Because testosterone stimulates bone formation and inhibits bone resorption that involve both androgen and estrogen

Table 3
Conditions associated with altered sex hormone-binding globulin concentrations

Increased SHBG	Decreased SHBG
HIV	Opioids
Liver disease	Androgens
Hyperthyroidism	Hypothyroidism
Estrogens	Nephrotic syndrome
Anticonvulsants	Glucocorticoids
Low testosterone	Acromegaly
Age (1%/year)	Obesity (IR)

Abbreviations: HIV, human immunodeficiency virus; SHBG, sex hormone-binding globulin.
From The Optimal evaluation of the infertile male: AUA best practice statement. American Urologic Association 2010. Available at: http://www.auanet.org/guidelines/male-infertility-optimal-evaluation-(reviewed-and-validity-confirmed-2011); with permission. Accessed May 21, 2017.

receptor-mediated processes, older men are at greater risk of low trauma fracture.[9–11] In men with severe androgen deficiency with or without low trauma fracture measurement of bone mineral density by dual-energy x-ray absorptiometry (DEXA) scanning is also recommended.[1,9]

TESTOSTERONE REPLACEMENT THERAPY

Testosterone replacement therapy (TRT) is indicated in men with primary or secondary hypogonadism. The goal of TRT is to treat the signs and symptoms of hypogonadism and achieve and maintain eugonadal serum testosterone levels. US Food and Drug Administration (FDA)-approved testosterone replacement treatments are numerous and varied in their route of administration and duration of action. The restrictive access to all currently available modalities is likely the result of the unprecedented surge in prescriptions for TRT. According to data from IMS Health, testosterone sales have increased 33% annually since 2012. Experts suggest that FDA scrutiny of TRT was rooted in the surge of TRT prescribed to men who have not undergone an appropriate evaluation when suspected of having testosterone deficiency.[12] Testosterone treatment modalities currently available in the United States include injectable (propionate, cypionate, enanthate, undecanoate), commercially available topical preparations (gels, patches, solution), implantable pellets, and oral or buccal forms (**Table 4**). The various preparations have varied durations of action and adverse reactions unique to the route of administration. Careful consideration must be taken to ensure the patient is compliant with the prescribed treatment regimen. Additionally, laboratory monitoring of the response to TRT and adverse reactions are also slightly different due to the modality being prescribed.

HYPOGONADISM AND PROSTATE CANCER

Use of TRT in men with prostate cancer remains controversial. Numerous studies have shown that TRT can decrease the overall mortality risk in hypogonadal men with or without prostate cancer. Historically, it has been widely accepted that testosterone may potentiate the growth of prostate cancer cells, resulting in the recommendation that TRT not be used or be used with extreme caution in men with a known diagnosis of prostate cancer regardless of treatment. However, recent data have provided evidence supporting that there is no increased risk of progression or recurrence of prostate cancer in men treated or untreated with a confirmed diagnosis of prostate cancer.[13,14] More recent data suggest that TRT may be safe in men with a known history of prostate cancer; however, researchers concluded that more studies are needed. Further evidence has shown low-serum testosterone levels have been associated with a greater risk of prostate cancer and a higher grade of disease.[15] Furthermore, the rate of prostate cancer progression and recurrence in men treated for prostate cancer tends to be lower in hypogonadal men treated with TRT than in those men not treated with TRT.[12] Recent data now suggest that TRT may be protective against the development and recurrence of prostate cancer. The prostate saturation model explains the changes in prostate-specific antigen in response to TRT and androgen deprivation therapy to treat prostate cancer.[15]

HYPOGONADISM AND CARDIOMETABOLIC SYNDROME

Testosterone deficiency has been shown to be associated with the following increased cardiovascular events and risk factors: dyslipidemia (eg, low high-density lipoprotein and elevated triglycerides), hypertension, obesity, diabetes mellitus, and

Table 4
Testosterone treatment modalities

		Topical or Transdermal		
Formulation	**Dosage**	**Adverse Effects**	**Benefits**	**Cons**
Androgel 1%, Androgel 1.62%, Testim, Fortesta	5–10 g/d	Skin irritation Transference	Maintain T level concentration over a 24-h period High patient adherence	Expensive, transference risk, drug accumulation, variable absorption, messy, daily administration
Transdermal Patch Androderm	2–4 mg patch qd	Skin irritation Transference	T levels mimic circadian rhythm Low incidence of polycythemia	Moderate cost, visible (not discreet), difficulty in maintaining adequate T concentration, skin irritation, lack of adhesiveness, daily administration
Topical Solution Axiron	60–120 mg applied to axilla qd	Skin irritation Transference	Maintain T levels over 24-h period Unique administration presumed to minimize risk of transference	Not yet known
		Buccal or Oral		
Formulation	**Dosage**	**Adverse Effects**	**Benefits**	**Cons**
Buccal System Striant	30 mg q 12 h	Alterations in taste and irritation of gums and oral mucosa	Testosterone levels within physiologic range	Moderate cost Oral irritation Twice-daily dosing
Fluoxymesterone Halotestin	5–40 mg daily	Hepatotoxicity	Pill form	See AE

Injectable

Formulation	Dosage	Adverse Effects	Benefits	Cons
Testosterone Cypionate Depo-Testosterone	50–400 mg IM q 10–14 d	Mood fluctuations or changes in libido, pain at injection site, excessive erythrocytosis	Effective in relieving symptoms, inexpensive	Supraphysiologic fluctuations, can be painful, requires OV q 10–14 d
Testosterone Enanthate Delatestryl	50–400 mg IM q wk	Mood fluctuations or changes in libido, pain at injection site, excessive erythrocytosis	Effective in relieving symptoms, inexpensive	Supraphysiologic fluctuations, can be painful, requires OV q wk
Testosterone Undecanoate Nebido[1], Aveed[2]	1000 mg IM q 6 wk during first 12 wk, then 1000 mg q 3 mo 750 mg IM initially, followed by 2nd injection 4 wk later, then q 10 wk (REMS certification required)	Mood fluctuations or changes in libido, pain at injection site, excessive erythrocytosis, pulmonary oil microembolism	Effective in relieving symptoms, inexpensive, long acting	Pain at injection site, cough and SOB

Implantable

Formulation	Dosage	Adverse Effects or Cons	Benefits
Testopel 75 mg pellets	6 pellets* implanted q 3–4 mo	Pain at insertion site, infection, expulsion, pain at insertion site, infection, expensive, requires OV	Long-acting, convenient, consistent delivery for a prolonged period of time

Abbreviations: AE, adverse event; IM, intramuscular; OV, office visit; REMS, risk evaluation mitigation strategy; SOB, shortness of breath.
* Medicare pellet limit per insertion.

insulin resistance. In addition, testosterone has an inverse relationship with BMI, waist circumference, low-density lipoprotein, and triglycerides.[16–19] However, it is not known whether hypogonadism is the cause of or the consequence of these conditions. Physiologically, it is understood that an increase in adiposity in men followed by aromatization of adipose tissue results in an increase in estradiol and adipokine production, leading to suppression of the hypothalamic pituitary secretion of LH, thus decreasing testosterone production by Leydig cells in the testicles. Furthermore, an increase in insulin resistance also occurs, which further inhibits Leydig cell production of testosterone.[19,20] Consequently, hypogonadal, obese patients with diabetes mellitus are at further risk of poor glycemic control, resulting in an increased risk of development of complications of diabetes and an increase in overall mortality risk. Recent studies have shown that testosterone therapy can ameliorate cardiometabolic risk. In a study conducted by the US Department of Veterans Affairs, researchers conducted an observational study to determine if TRT improved overall mortality. The data showed that over a 4-year period overall mortality decreased by 10.3% in the treated group and 20.7% in the untreated group.[21] In men with type II diabetes, researchers showed that over a 6-year period all-cause mortality was 19.2% in untreated men and 8.4% in men treated with TRT.[22]

DISCUSSION

The increased prevalence of hypogonadism and subsequent surge in treatment has forced experts to establish effective guidelines for the evaluation and treatment of hypogonadism. Physician assistants (PAs) caring for these patients must be able to accurately diagnose, treat, and manage these patients effectively. The International Society for Sexual Medicine (ISSM) guidelines provide the most comprehensive and current data pertinent to patients who are more likely to present to a urology practice.[3] The ISSM guidelines contain information and guidance regarding patients with urologic disease, including recommendations for patients with prostate cancer and benign prostatic hypertrophy. The ISSM guidelines also address the controversy surrounding cardiovascular risk associated with TRT. Experts reviewed the literature in search of evidence to support the claim that TRT increases cardiovascular risk and their findings indicate there were no studies conducted that produced evidence to support that claim. The data discovered by the researchers indicated that TRT in hypogonadal men actually decreased the risk of cardiovascular disease.[3,23] Researchers further concluded that randomized controlled trials will be critical to accurately determine the efficacy and safety of TRT with or without significant comorbidities.

SOCIETAL ISSUES

Societal pressure and widespread advertising have also contributed to men inappropriately seeking treatment of hypogonadism. In cities across the nation, so-called Low T centers have been established to treat men with presumed hypogonadism. Many of these establishments provide suboptimal evaluations and often initiate inappropriate treatment, which often leads to adverse reactions. Clear communication between the clinician and the patient is paramount to dispelling inaccurate information or advertised promises that lead patients to have unrealistic expectations about the benefits of TRT. Further clarification is important for both the clinician and the patient to understand the difference between testosterone supplementation and TRT. Testosterone supplementation involves the addition of testosterone in cases in which the levels of testosterone are already in the normal range. This practice is typically done by bodybuilders or athletes to increase muscle mass, whereas testosterone replacement is the act of restoring abnormally low or deficient testosterone levels back into the normal range. Patient counseling defining these terms and the expected treatment outcomes is essential to helping the patient understand the true benefits of TRT while setting realistic expectations. PAs should also counsel patients with hypogonadism to make appropriate lifestyle modifications that support normal androgen production and/or improve response to therapy. Improving nutrition, increasing exercise, and decreasing or discontinuing medications contributing to the patient's hypogonadism will also support improvement in endogenous testosterone production and symptom relief.

SUMMARY

Effective evaluation, treatment, and management of hypogonadism in a clinical practice will be best conducted by adhering to the various published guidelines and understanding which approach would be best suited for appropriately diagnosing and managing men with hypogonadism. PAs in a primary care practice must also be abreast of current recommendations for hypogonadal men with a diagnosis of prostate cancer when considering treatment. Being aware of and understanding the various associated comorbidities with hypogonadism will help clinicians positively affect the overall health and well-being of these patients. Remaining aware of and understanding the societal impact on the desire of men to seek treatment of hypogonadism will further help differentiate patients seeking testosterone supplementation rather than TRT. PAs using a consistent evidence-based approach for the treatment of hypogonadism can, it is hoped, contribute to the development of a singular and more widely accepted set of guidelines that would be beneficial to the evaluation, treatment, and management of hypogonadal men.

REFERENCES

1. Bhasin S, Cunningham GR, Hayes FJ, et al, Task Force, Endocrine Society. Testosterone therapy in men with androgen deficiency syndromes: Endocrine Society clinical practice guideline. J Clin Endocrinol Metab 2010;95(6):2536–59.
2. Mulligan T, Frick M, Zuraw Q, et al. Prevalence of hypogonadism in males aged at least 45 years: the HIM study. Int J Clin Pract 2006;60(7):762–9.
3. Dean JD, McMahon CG, Guay AT, et al. The International Society for Sexual Medicine's process of care for the assessment and management of testosterone deficiency in adult men. J Sex Med 2015;12(8):1660–86.
4. AACE Hypogonadism Task Force. American Association of Clinical Endocrinologists medical guidelines for clinical practice for the evaluation and treatment of hypogonadism in adult male patients—2002 update. Endocr Pract 2002;8(6):439–56.
5. Svartberg J, von Mühlen D, Sundsfjord J, et al. Waist circumference and testosterone levels in community dwelling men: the Tromsø study. Eur J Epidemiol 2004;19(7):657–63.
6. Handelsman DJ, Liu PY. "Klinefelter's syndrome—a microcosm of male reproductive health." J Clin Endocrinol Metab 2006;91:1220–2.
7. The Optimal Evaluation of the Infertile Male: AUA best practice statement. American Urological Association 2010. Available at: http://www.auanet.org/guidelines/male-infertility-optimal-evaluation-(reviewed-and-validity-confirmed-2011). Accessed May 21, 2017.
8. Wang C, Nieschlag E, Swerdloff R, et al. Investigation, treatment and monitoring of late-onset hypogonadism in males. Int J Androl 2009;32:1–10.

9. Mascarenhas MR, et al. Effects of male hypogonadism treatment on the bone mineral density. 2017.

10. Jackson JA, et al. Estradiol, testosterone, and the risk for hip fractures in elderly men from the Framingham study. Am J Med Sci 1992;304(1):4–8.

11. Ebeling PR. Osteoporosis in men. N Engl J Med 2008;358(14):1474–82.

12. Khera M. "Testosterone replacement therapy: controversies versus reality" grand rounds in urology. November 15, 2015. Available at: http://www.grandroundsinurology.com/TRT-Mohit-Khera-testosterone-replacement-therapy-controversies-versus-reality/. Accessed June 27, 2017.

13. Khera M, Grober ED, Najari B, et al. Testosterone replacement therapy following radical prostatectomy. J Sex Med 2009;6(4):1165–70.

14. Kaplan AL, Lenis AT, Shah A, et al. Testosterone replacement therapy in men with prostate cancer: a time-varying analysis. J Sex Med 2015;12(2):374–80.

15. Schatzl G, Madersbacher S, Thurridl T, et al. High-grade prostate cancer is associated with low serum testosterone levels. Prostate 2001;47(1):52–8.

16. Shabsigh R, Katz M, Yan G, et al. Cardiovascular issues in hypogonadism and testosterone therapy. Am J Cardiol 2005;96(12B):67M–72M.

17. Nettleship J, et al. "Testosterone and coronary artery disease." Advances in the management of testosterone deficiency, vol. 37. Karger Publishers; 2009. p. 91–107.

18. Page ST, Mohr BA, Link CL, et al. Higher testosterone levels are associated with increased high-density lipoprotein cholesterol in men with cardiovascular disease: results from the Massachusetts Male Aging Study. Asian J Androl 2008; 10(2):193–200.

19. Aso Y. Cardiovascular disease in patients with diabetic nephropathy. Curr Mol Med 2008;8(6):533–43.

20. Kapoor D, Malkin CJ, Channer KS, et al. Androgens, insulin resistance and vascular disease in men. Clin Endocrinol 2005;63(3):239–50.

21. Shores MM, Smith NL, Forsberg CW, et al. Testosterone treatment and mortality in men with low testosterone levels. J Clin Endocrinol Metab 2012;97(6):2050–8.

22. Muraleedharan V, Marsh H, Kapoor D, et al. Testosterone deficiency is associated with increased risk of mortality and testosterone replacement improves survival in men with type 2 diabetes. Eur J Endocrinol 2013;169(6):725–33.

23. Morgentaler A, Miner MM, Caliber M, et al. Testosterone therapy and cardiovascular risk: advances and controversies. Mayo Clin Proc 2015;90(2):224–51.

Male Infertility

Mark C. Lindgren, MD

KEYWORDS

- Male • Infertility • Semen analysis • Azoospermia • Oligospermia • Hypogonadism
- Testosterone • Klinefelter syndrome

KEY POINTS

- A male factor contribution to infertility is common. Ten percent to 15% of all couples attempting to conceive are infertile and half of these infertile couples have a male factor contribution.
- The proper initial workup for male factor infertility requires a thorough medical history, including medication use, and complete physical examination, including genitalia, serum laboratory testing, and at least 2 complete semen analyses.
- Exogenous testosterone usage is a common modern cause or contributor to male infertility and can have a lasting impact on a man's fertility potential.

INTRODUCTION

Infertility is defined as the inability to achieve pregnancy after 1 year of regular, unprotected intercourse. Infertility is a disease, in that it is a deviation from the normal function of a body part, organ, or system, in this case, the reproductive system.[1] Ten percent to 15% of all couples suffer from infertility, regardless of race, culture, or ethnicity.[2] In the absence of testing, infertility is a disease of couples. With testing, approximately 20% of couples are found to have both male and female factors that contribute to their infertility. In an additional 30% of couples, a significant male factor is the lone cause. Therefore, 50% of all infertile couples have a male factor contribution to problem.[3] Infertility is a significant stressor in the lives of both the male and female partners that can strain relationships and lead to separation and divorce.[4] The financial burden for infertility treatments, such as cycles of in vitro fertilization with intracytoplasmic sperm injection (IVF/ICSI), which are often not covered by insurance, can easily reach into the tens of thousands of dollars. This out-of-pocket expense can be a significant financial stressor to some and prohibitively expensive for others. The workup and treatment of male factor infertility can offer, in many cases, a cost-effective means to achieve healthy pregnancies without the need for IVF/ICSI.[5]

Disclosures: The author has nothing to disclose.
Department of Urology, The University of Oklahoma, 920 Stanton L Young Boulevard, WP 3150, Oklahoma City, OK 73104, USA
E-mail address: Mark-Lindgren@ouhsc.edu

Physician Assist Clin 3 (2018) 139–147
http://dx.doi.org/10.1016/j.cpha.2017.08.002

Furthermore, male factor infertility can be a sign of a different, potentially life-threatening disease, such as testis cancer, that would be discovered only on physical examination, which is part of a standard infertility workup.[6] Because of this, male factor infertility always deserves, at the very least, a complete initial workup, which is described in detail as follows.

EVALUATION OF THE MALE

Any couple with a female partner younger than 35 years that meets the definition of infertility (12 months of regular, unprotected intercourse without pregnancy) warrants further study. Couples in which the female partner is 35 or older, should consider evaluation after 6 months without pregnancy due to diminished fecundity of the woman beyond the age of 35. Additionally, if a couple presents with any known male or female risk factors or concerns, they can undergo evaluation without a requisite infertile timeframe or even before attempting conception. Couples seeking a fertility workup always should be offered simultaneous evaluation of the man and woman, the man being the focus of this article.[1] The basic evaluation of the infertile man includes a medical history, physical examination, 2 complete semen analyses, and hormonal serum laboratory testing, all of which are covered within this text.

HISTORY

A thorough medical history is important to identify possible risk factors for infertility in men, and always should begin with a reproductive history. The duration of time without conception is a defining factor of infertility and necessary to determine if the diagnosis is applicable. Infertility is further subdivided into primary and secondary infertility. If the patient has never achieved pregnancy with any partner at any time, this is referred to as primary infertility, whereas patients who have had prior conceptions or children with either the current or a previous partner and are currently infertile are suffering from secondary infertility. Determining if a man has secondary infertility can help narrow the differential diagnosis if he successfully fathered children in the past.[7]

Timing of intercourse is also an important historical component. Ideally, couples should have intercourse either daily or every other day around the time of ovulation. For a woman with regular periods, ovulation occurs approximately 14 days before the onset of menses.[8] Couples can target the time of ovulation by marking a calendar or by using various modern apps that help track female cycles. Ovulation can be more precisely targeted by basal body temperature monitoring, transvaginal ultrasounds, serum hormone testing, or, most commonly, ovulation prediction kits. Ovulation prediction kits are widely available at drug stores and simply require urinating onto the testing device, much like a home pregnancy test. For couples that have not been timing intercourse around ovulation, it is important to determine the frequency of sex. Couples that have sex 3 to 4 times a week will definitely have sperm present during ovulation. However, couples that have sex once or twice a month could easily miss multiple ovulations over time.

A complete sexual history should always include erectile function, ejaculatory and orgasmic function, and history of lubricant usage. Erections satisfactory for penetrative intercourse and antegrade ejaculation are necessary for successful reproduction. On the other hand, dysfunction of erections or ejaculation can be indicative of additional pathology, hormonal or otherwise. Curvature of the erect penis, either due to Peyronie disease or congenital curvature, can interfere with successful intercourse and the deposition of sperm in the vaginal vault. Although lubricants can help facilitate sex for many couples, most commercial sexual lubricants adversely affect sperm mobility, and some are specifically designed to be spermicidal. There are commercially available lubricants based on hydroxyethylcellulose that specifically do not impair or minimally impair sperm, such as Pre-Seed (INGfertility, Spokane, WA) and ConceivEase (Reproductive Laboratory, Memphis, TN).[9] However, it is best for couples to avoid lubricants, if possible, or use a safer variety of lubricant sparingly, if necessary.

Several risk factors for infertility can be discovered from the patient's childhood history. Bilateral cryptorchidism and subsequent orchiopexy is sometimes known by the patient or can be suspected on physical examination.[10] Testicular torsion or testicular trauma requiring medical attention is often a pediatric or adolescent-aged event and usually quite memorable to the patient. If the presence of a varicocele is known, patients usually offer this information early in the history given its association with infertility. Either precocious or delayed puberty, and problems with sexual development have a variety of etiologies, which are important to determine. All of these conditions, which may be elicited from the patient's childhood history, are associated with impaired spermatogenesis and male infertility.

A patient's further medical and surgical history can reveal a variety of risk factors. History of sexually transmitted disease, urinary tract infection, prostatitis, and epididymitis can be related to obstructed or impaired sperm transport. Mumps orchitis, although relatively rare in the United States, can significantly damage testicular function when it occurs during or after puberty. Spermatogenesis takes place over 2 to 3 months, and any recent febrile illness can significantly impair spermatogenesis for a similar period of months. Poorly controlled diabetes mellitus and neurologic pathologies, such as spinal cord injury or multiple sclerosis, can cause erectile and ejaculatory dysfunction. Similarly, retroperitoneal and pelvic surgery can directly damage the nerves critical for proper ejaculation. Chemotherapy, radiation therapy, and stem cell transplantation can render a patient temporarily or permanently sterile.

A variety of medications, environmental toxins, and recreational drugs impair a man's fertility either by disrupting his endocrine system, by impairing the mechanical transport of sperm, or by direct toxicity to the testis and spermatogenesis. These medications include gonadotropin-releasing hormone agonists/antagonists, alpha-blockers, various antibiotics, sulfasalazine, cimetidine, spironolactone, calcium channel blockers, colchicine, opioids, and a variety of psychiatric drugs. Environmental or work exposure to heavy metals, pesticides, phthalates, and some other industrial chemicals are known to impair fertility. Heavy alcohol use, tobacco, marijuana, and cocaine have all been shown to impair semen parameters. Exogenous testosterone, an increasingly common medication, is a fairly effective contraceptive. Men taking testosterone and concerned about current or future fertility are addressed more thoroughly later in this article.

PHYSICAL EXAMINATION

For the average infertile man, the most important portion of the physical is the scrotal examination, but all examinations should begin more generally. Key features to note include body habitus and obesity, gynecoid, body hair, gynecomastia, degree of virilization, male pattern balding, and Tanner stage. These general findings, if present, can be related to endocrine dysfunction and/or genetic abnormalities.

Examination of the phallus includes location of the urethral meatus, orthotopic or hypospadic, penile size being normal or microphallic, whether the penis is buried in subcutaneous fat, the presence of flaccid curvature, and lesions present. Testicular volume should be measured by either calipers or Prader orchidometer. Normal testicular size is greater than or equal to 4 cm in the long axis by caliper measurement or

20 mL by orchidometer volume measurement. Most testicular volume is dedicated to spermatogenesis. Likewise, decreased testicular size is associated with impaired spermatogenesis.[11] Testicular consistency should be noted, be it firm or soft, as well as a careful examination for any testicular masses. The left and right epididymis are palpated and the presence of caput, corpus, and cauda verified as well as continuity with the vas deferens. The quality of the epididymides should be soft, as induration can be consistent with a downstream obstructive process. Careful palpation of the vasa is also necessary to confirm the absence of atretic regions consistent with congenital obstruction.

Varicoceles are an abnormal dilatation of the spermatic veins, which have a characteristic "bag of worms" quality on palpation. Varicoceles cause progressive damage to the testicles and their spermatogenic potential over time. The damage is thought to be largely due to a thermal effect, whereby the dilated spermatic veins disrupt the cooling mechanism of the testes and result in loss of function.[12] Assessment for varicoceles requires evaluation in the standing position at rest as well as during Valsalva. Grade III varicoceles are visible through the scrotal skin at rest, grade II are palpable at rest, and grade I varicoceles are palpable only during Valsalva. All varicoceles should enlarge during Valsalva and diminish on lying down. Varicoceles that do not collapse with the patient supine are concerning for other possible pelvic or abdominal pathology and may warrant imaging. Most varicoceles do not require further evaluation with scrotal ultrasound, but some patients who are difficult to examine due to a contracted scrotum or enlarged habitus may benefit from ultrasound evaluation. Varicoceles are an important modifiable cause for impaired spermatogenesis. With a simple outpatient surgery to repair a unilateral or bilateral varicocele, patients can have improved semen parameters, increased pregnancy rates via intercourse, and increased success rates of intrauterine insemination, as well as IVF/ICSI.[13–15]

Routine Serum Laboratory Testing

At a minimum, serum total testosterone and follicle stimulating hormone (FSH) are needed for initial evaluation of the infertile male. Additionally, many male infertility specialists, including the author, routinely obtain luteinizing hormone (LH) and estradiol at initial evaluation. A borderline testosterone may warrant retesting of total testosterone in conjunction with albumin and sex hormone binding globulin (SHBG) to determine the bioavailable testosterone. Serum testosterone, albumin, and SHBG measurements can be used to determine bioavailable testosterone via an algorithm that is freely available on multiple online Web sites.[16] Circulating testosterone is found in 3 states in the serum: free or unbound, loosely bound to albumin, and tightly bound to SHBG. The bioavailable testosterone represents the amount of free and loosely bound testosterone that is available to diffuse into the cell and activate the androgen receptor. Laboratory assays that attempt to directly measure free testosterone are notoriously inaccurate and discouraged from routine use. A low serum testosterone measurement may prompt further testing of serum prolactin or imaging of the pituitary gland, but neither should be routinely ordered.

SEMEN ANALYSIS

Perhaps the most important test to determine a man's potential fertility is the semen analysis. A minimum of 2 specimens collected at least 2 to 4 weeks apart are required for initial evaluation due to the variability of any individual's semen parameters. It is important to verify that the laboratory is using the current methodology for semen analysis, which would be reflected in the report by the proper reference values for the semen parameters. At the writing of this article, the current World Health Organization reference values are the fifth edition, 2010 standards[17]:

- Semen volume $\geq$1.5 mL
- Concentration greater than 15 million sperm/mL
- Total sperm count greater than 39 million sperm
- Total motility greater than 40%
- Kruger strict morphology greater than 4%

Verify the period of abstinence before the semen analysis was, at a minimum, 48 hours since the patient last ejaculated, and no more than 7 days since the last ejaculation. Semen analyses are ideally collected by masturbation in a private collection room within the laboratory facility and then analyzed immediately on collection. If collection must be performed at home, the sample should be transported to the laboratory and evaluated as soon as possible, as sperm start to die and become immotile in the collection cup. In addition to the reference values listed previously, complete semen analyses should include pH, days abstinent, numerical assessment of sperm progression, and quantification of round cells or white blood cells (WBCs), if present. Round cells within a semen analysis are most likely to be either immature spermatocytes or WBCs, but cannot be differentiated by microscopy. A WBC assay is necessary to determine the presence of WBCs, which indicates possible inflammation or infection in the genitourinary tract or organs, and may necessitate further testing, such as semen culture. If the motility is significantly low, laboratories should also perform and document the results of vitality staining.[17]

PROPER REFERRAL

Infertile men should all undergo the basic workup as described previously, including history, physical examination, hormone testing and semen analyses. Any abnormality of semen parameters and/or serum hormones warrants referral to a reproductive urologist, the specialist dedicated to managing problems with fertility in men. Sexual or ejaculatory dysfunction, depending on the problem, is managed by most general urologists as well as primary care physicians. Any abnormal examination findings of the genitalia also may warrant referral to a urologist.

FURTHER TESTING

Digital rectal examination (DRE) is not routinely indicated for the infertile male, but should be offered for any male who either complains of lower urinary tract symptoms or is old enough to warrant prostate cancer screening. For the purpose of infertility, DREs are performed if ejaculatory duct obstruction is suspected. An azoospermic semen analysis, with low volume (<1.5 mL), and a relatively acidic pH (<7.2) is suspicious for possible ejaculatory duct obstruction. Normally, the seminal vesicle contribution to the seminal fluid has a basic pH and represents more than 60% of the volume. When the ejaculatory ducts are obstructed, the seminal vesicle portion as well as the sperm are blocked, and the semen produced comes primarily from the smaller volume contribution made by the prostate, which is more acidic. If ejaculatory duct obstruction is suspected, a DRE can be performed to evaluate for dilation of the seminal vesicles or the presence of a midline cyst. However, transrectal ultrasound is the gold standard test to evaluate this condition and should be performed regardless of DRE findings.

Scrotal ultrasound is recommended only in patients with difficult or inadequate scrotal examinations, or to better visualize ambiguous findings. Scrotal/inguinal ultrasound, when used to detect varicoceles, must be performed in standing position both with and without Valsalva. Some institutions have special orders for varicocele evaluation by ultrasound, otherwise this should be explicitly written in the order's comments.

Patients with congenital bilateral absence of the vas deferens (CBAVD) are azoospermic and easily identified during scrotal examination. Up to 80% of these men also have mutations of the cystic fibrosis transmembrane conductance regulator (CFTR) gene, which makes them carriers of cystic fibrosis. Both male and female individuals should undergo CFTR gene testing when CBAVD is found before any attempts at reproduction via in vitro fertilization due to the risk of their offspring either becoming a carrier (50% risk) or being afflicted with cystic fibrosis (25% risk).

Patients with a unilaterally absent vas deferens have a high incidence of renal agenesis on the ipsilateral side. This association is due to the influence that the Wolffian ducts, part of which become the vasa, have on renal development in utero. Any patient found to have an absent vas deferens should undergo renal ultrasonography to determine if both kidneys are present. Additionally, there is a lesser association between patients with CBAVD and patients with renal agenesis. Patients with CBAVD should be offered a renal ultrasound only if their CFTR testing is negative.

Patients found to be azoospermic or severely oligospermic (<5 million sperm/mL) should have karyotype testing performed, which simply requires a peripheral blood draw. The potential outcomes of karyotyping are too numerous to cover within this article. One common abnormal finding in the infertile male is a 47, XXY karyotype, consistent with Klinefelter syndrome, covered in further detail later in this article. In addition to a full karyotype, specific regions on the Y chromosome are associated with azoospermia and have been identified as critical for normal sperm production. These portions of the Y chromosome are appropriately named as Azoospermia Factor or AZF regions a, b, and c. If microdeletions are detected within AZFa or AZFb, the patient is, unfortunately, not able to produce sperm whatsoever, and should be counseled to pursue donor sperm or adoption. Patients with microdeletions involving only the AZFc region have been found to have a low level of spermatogenesis, which may be found during microsurgical testicular sperm extraction. Y chromosome microdeletion testing is recommended for azoospermic patients and previously routinely ordered for all severely oligospermic patients.

A wide variety of advanced sperm testing exists and has been studied throughout the years. These tests include DNA fragmentation assays, fluorescence in situ hybridization testing, sperm penetration assays, postcoital mucus testing, acrosome reaction testing, anti-sperm antibody assays, and reactive oxygen species assays. Although these studies have advanced our knowledge of sperm function and dysfunction, most of these advanced tests have a limited role in clinical medicine. The utility of these tests, or lack thereof, are best discussed with one's local reproductive endocrinologists, the female reproductive specialists, before ordering. Often the information gained from these tests does not change clinical management and can simply leave the patient with an uncovered, unwanted laboratory bill.

Klinefelter Syndrome: 47, XXY

Patients with Klinefelter syndrome are typically azoospermic; undervirilized; have small, firm testes; low serum testosterone; disproportionately long limbs on examination; and potentially gynecomastia. Approximately 10% of patients presenting with nonobstructive azoospermia have Klinefelter syndrome, making it the most common genetic cause of nonobstructive azoospermia. The syndrome often occurs due to a nondisjunction event in either the paternal or maternal gamete during meiosis, which results in an extra

X chromosome. However, mosaicism of 46, XY and 47, XXY has been noted in patients, which is likely due to a nondisjunction event during mitosis in the embryo. Despite azoospermia in semen analyses, more than 60% of patients with Klinefelter syndrome are found to have a low level of spermatogenesis during microsurgical sperm extraction. This is thought to be due to that same mosaicism within the germ cells: the 47, XXY germ cells do not produce sperm, but 46, XY germ cells produce sperm, which can be used for in vitro fertilization. Nevertheless, it is recommended that couples using surgically extracted sperm have their embryos undergo preimplantation genetic testing to limit the risk of Klinefelter syndrome to the offspring.

EXOGENOUS TESTOSTERONE

The treatment of symptomatic hypogonadism has increased greatly over the past decade due to the variety of testosterone formulations available, the marketing efforts of large pharmaceutical companies, and the pervasive community men's health clinics that are multiplying throughout our cities. Ten percent to 12% of documented testosterone prescriptions are written for men younger than 40 years, the traditional age of reproduction. Furthermore, men, much like women, are more commonly delaying reproduction until later in life. Unfortunately, these men receiving testosterone may not be appropriately counseled regarding its effects on fertility. Testosterone is a fairly effective male contraceptive that shuts down spermatogenesis in many patients and can cause a long-lasting or permanent decrease in testicular function. This can certainly be counterintuitive to the naïve patient who may feel especially virile as he experiences increased vitality, libido, and sexual function. That same patient may be quite confused when he is unable to achieve pregnancy and subsequently finds his sperm counts are quite low or zero. These patients are becoming increasingly common in infertility clinics; one study found that 7% of men presenting for infertility had been on exogenous testosterone therapy. Unfortunately, many well-meaning physicians do not necessarily understand these implications.[18] An infamous survey of the members of the American Urologic Association in 2010, found that up to 25% of respondents would actually treat hypogonadal, infertile men with testosterone while actively pursuing pregnancy, thereby potentially compounding the problem.

The reason exogenous testosterone is damaging to a man's fertility potential is due to the regulation and negative feedback vital for testicular function. The 2 main functions of the testis, spermatogenesis and testosterone production, are entirely dependent on stimulation via the pituitary hormones, FSH and LH, respectively. When exogenous testosterone is present, the negative feedback mechanism, via the hypothalamus and pituitary, determines there is plenty of testosterone in the system. Almost universally, the serum levels of FSH and LH appropriately drop to undetectable or near-zero levels. Without FSH and LH stimulation, the testicles appropriately shut down spermatogenesis and endogenous testosterone production. Over time, the testicles can slowly atrophy and have decreased recovery potential with cessation of testosterone.

Patients who present with infertility and exogenous testosterone use, should first and foremost, stop the exogenous testosterone. A recent study by Kohn and colleagues,[19] showed recovery of even a low level of spermatogenesis can take 6, 12, or even 24 months after cessation of testosterone, and is not a guarantee. Recovery is seen more readily in younger men who have taken testosterone for shorter periods. Hypogonadism itself, even without exposure to exogenous testosterone, is related to decreased spermatogenesis. The spermatogenic potential of these patients at baseline, before exposure, is usually unknown.

Studies of testosterone as a potential contraceptive were performed decades ago on healthy, eugonadal men with normal sperm counts and normal testosterone. In one such study, after 18 months of exogenous testosterone, 70% of men appropriately developed azoospermia or severe oligozoospermia, but only 85% of those men regained sperm counts to a reasonable level on cessation. A similar study found that with cessation of testosterone after only 6 months, only 46% of men achieved their baseline semen parameters. Recovery of spermatogenesis can be aided by medications, such as clomiphene citrate and human chorionic gonadotropin, but it is recommended that complex fertility and hormone management should be referred to a reproductive urology specialist.

REFERENCES

1. Practice Committee of American Society for Reproductive Medicine. Definitions of infertility and recurrent pregnancy loss: a committee opinion. Fertil Steril 2013;99(1):63.
2. Stephen EH, Chandra A. Declining estimates of infertility in the United States: 1982-2002. Fertil Steril 2006;86(3):516–23.
3. Thonneau P, Marchand S, Tallec A, et al. Incidence and main causes of infertility in a resident population (1,850,000) of three French regions (1988-1989). Hum Reprod 1991;6(6):811–6.
4. Valsangkar S, Bodhare T, Bele S, et al. An evaluation of the effect of infertility on marital, sexual satisfaction indices and health-related quality of life in women. J Hum Reprod Sci 2011;4(2):80–5.
5. Schlegel PN. Is assisted reproduction the optimal treatment for varicocele-associated male infertility? a cost-effectiveness analysis. Urology 1997;49(1): 83–90.
6. Honig SC, Lipshultz LI, Jarow J. Significant medical pathology uncovered by a comprehensive male infertility evaluation. Fertil Steril 1994;62(5):1028–34.
7. Practice Committee of American Society for Reproductive Medicine. Diagnostic evaluation of the infertile male: a committee opinion. Fertil Steril 2015;103(3): e18–25.
8. Practice Committee of American Society for Reproductive Medicine in collaboration with Society for Reproductive Endocrinology and Infertility. Optimizing natural fertility: a committee opinion. Fertil Steril 2013;100(3):631–7.
9. Agarwal A, Deepinder F, Cocuzza M, et al. Effect of vaginal lubricants on sperm motility and chromatin integrity: a prospective comparative study. Fertil Steril 2008;89(2):375–9.
10. Murphy F, Paran TS, Puri P. Orchidopexy and its impact on fertility. Pediatr Surg Int 2007;23(7):625–32.
11. Lipshultz LI, Corriere JN Jr. Progressive testicular atrophy in the varicocele patient. J Urol 1977;117(2):175–6.
12. Chehval MJ, Purcell MH. Deterioration of semen parameters over time in men with untreated varicocele: evidence of progressive testicular damage. Fertil Steril 1992;57(1):174–7.
13. Kim ED, Leibman BB, Grinblat DM, et al. Varicocele repair improves semen parameters in azoospermic men with spermatogenic failure. J Urol 1999;162(3 Pt 1): 737–40.
14. Matthews GJ, Matthews ED, Goldstein M. Induction of spermatogenesis and achievement of pregnancy after microsurgical varicocelectomy in men with azoospermia and severe oligoasthenospermia. Fertil Steril 1998;70(1):71–5.

15. Kirby EW, Wiener LE, Rajanahally S, et al. Undergoing varicocele repair before assisted reproduction improves pregnancy rate and live birth rate in azoospermic and oligospermic men with a varicocele: a systematic review and meta-analysis. Fertil Steril 2016;106(6):1338–43.
16. Vermeulen A, Verdonck L, Kaufman JM. A critical evaluation of simple methods for the estimation of free testosterone in serum. J Clin Endocrinol Metab 1999; 84(10):3666–72.
17. Jequier AM. Semen analysis: a new manual and its application to the understanding of semen and its pathology. Asian J Androl 2010;12(1):11–3.
18. Kolettis PN, Purcell ML, Parker W, et al. Medical testosterone: an iatrogenic cause of male infertility and a growing problem. Urology 2015;85:1068–73.
19. Kohn TP, Louis MR, Pickett SM, et al. Age and duration of testosterone therapy predict time to return of sperm count after human chorionic gonadotropin therapy. Fertil Steril 2017;107(2):351–7.e1.

Moving?

Make sure your subscription moves with you!

To notify us of your new address, find your **Clinics Account Number** (located on your mailing label above your name), and contact customer service at:

Email: journalscustomerservice-usa@elsevier.com

800-654-2452 (subscribers in the U.S. & Canada)
314-447-8871 (subscribers outside of the U.S. & Canada)

Fax number: 314-447-8029

Elsevier Health Sciences Division
Subscription Customer Service
3251 Riverport Lane
Maryland Heights, MO 63043

*To ensure uninterrupted delivery of your subscription, please notify us at least 4 weeks in advance of move.